Preface

SCOPME began its work on continuing professional development in 1993 and this resulted in the publication of two working papers in 1994 and 1998.

Following discussions with the NHSE, the Committee decided to undertake a further enquiry and, prior to the disbandment of SCOPME in March 1999, it was agreed that a report of this further work should be published.

The enquiry on which this report is based took place largely during 1998. Publication of this document has been delayed because of the need to put in hand arrangements to wind up the work of the Committee.

Since that time, other developments have taken place. The General Medical Council has published important proposals for the revalidation of specialists and general practitioners on which SCOPME has already commented in its document *The need for a process of review.* These are now being refined through a process of consultation. The Department of Health has published a further document in its series on quality in the new NHS *Continuing professional development: Quality in the new NHS,* July 1999.

The recommendations made by SCOPME in this its final report should be considered in the light of these other developments.

Contents

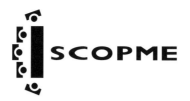

SCOPME

**THE STANDING COMMITTEE ON
POSTGRADUATE MEDICAL AND DENTAL EDUCATION**

A strategy for continuing education and professional development for hospital doctors and dentists

Including the research report:
Giving credit where credit is due
by Soundings Research

A SCOPME report   **1999**

About SCOPME

SCOPME was set up in August 1988 and was disbanded in March 1999 by Ministerial decision. It was concerned only with postgraduate and continuing medical and dental education in England.

SCOPME's terms of reference were to:
- Advise the Secretary of State on the delivery of postgraduate medical and dental education, taking into account both the standards promulgated by professional bodies and the potential difficulties of reconciling service and training needs;
- Identify particular problems and to develop realistic solutions to these in consultation with relevant interests;
- Report regularly.

Membership of SCOPME

Members of the Committee were appointed by the Secretary of State for Health on advice from the Chief Medical Officer and the Chief Dental Officer. Membership covered a wide range of educational, professional and service interests and the major bodies concerned are asked for advice in suggesting suitable names. Members of SCOPME were not expected to act as representatives of other bodies, but were appointed because of their individual expertise.

Acknowledgements

Scopme is indebted to the members of the steering group on continuing professional development, to Soundings Research, to those who participated in the workshop on CPD, and to all those who contributed to the Committee's discussions on this topic.

Publication notice

Copyright of this publication is held by the Department of Health. Further copying and distribution is permitted and encouraged for non-profit, educational purposes by those to whom it has been distributed. Summaries of selected SCOPME reports are available on the WorldWide Web at http://www.scopme.org.uk and recent reports can be downloaded.

There are three ways in which you can order copies of this publication:
- Telephone: NHS Responseline   0541 555 455   ● Fax: 01623 724 524
- Mail: Department of Health, PO Box 777, London SE1 6XH.

Production	
Editor	Jolyon Oxley
Copy editor and DTP	Ros Kenn
Management	John Egan
Editorial assistants	Barbara Baum and Jeannie Corrigan
Cover design	Tactica Solutions
Printed by	Tactica Solutions
Published by	The Standing Committee on Postgraduate Medical and Dental Education ©1999
ISBN	**1 873436 37 8**

1 The scope of this enquiry and recommendations

Since early 1993, SCOPME conducted a series of enquiries into the professional development needs of career grade doctors and dentists. A working paper published in 1994[1] was one of the initiatives that established the concept of continuing professional development (CPD) for all doctors and dentists. This was followed in 1998 by a second working paper[2] defining the nature and scope of CPD and its relationship to continuing medical education (CME), and making a series of recommendations concerning the CPD of hospital consultants. It also put forward some draft principles that might apply to CPD for all doctors and dentists. SCOPME considered that CME was largely concerned with clinical, specialty-based issues, whereas CPD was a broader process which assists clinicians in:

- Achieving personal and professional growth;
- Keeping abreast of, and managing, clinical, organisational and social changes that affect professional roles in general;
- Widening, developing and changing their own roles and responsibilities;
- Acquiring and refining the skills needed for new roles and responsibilities or career development;
- Putting individual development and learning needs into a team and multiprofessional context.

CPD has been featured and promoted by the Department of Health as a major component of clinical governance in its consultative document *A first class service: quality in the new NHS*.[3] SCOPME welcomed this initiative but cautioned that the White Paper's view of CPD was limited, and that there was a need for a widespread change of culture concerning the balance between the service needs of NHS trusts as employers, and the learning opportunities for the doctors and dentists whom they employ.

[More recently the NHS Executive has published a report which sets out a long-term vision for CPD and its role in supporting quality in the NHS. This document *Continuing Professional Development: Quality in the new NHS* has been issued with the Health Service Circular HSC 1999/154, dated 16 July 1999.]

Scope of SCOPME's further enquiries

Following a request from NHSE in 1996, SCOPME decided to undertake further work in the area of CPD and CME, with the intention of developing an educationally effective and affordable strategy for both processes. A steering group was established to oversee a programme of work which, from the outset, confirmed the previous SCOPME tenet that although CME was an important process in itself, it was nevertheless a substantial component of CPD rather than a separate entity.

References
1. SCOPME. *Continuing professional development for doctors and dentists*. 1994.
2. SCOPME. *Continuing professional development for doctors and dentists. Recommendations for hospital consultant CPD and draft principles for all doctors and dentists*. 1998.
3. Department of Health. *A first class service: quality in the new NHS*. 1998.

The steering group planned and supervised a programme of work in its attempt to devise a workable strategy for CME and CPD. This comprised:

1. An examination of the current expenditure on CME and CPD. A report of this work by Dr Annabelle Baughan was submitted to the Secretary of State in August 1997. The main finding was extreme variability in:
   - The ways that expenditure is recorded;
   - The ways that available funds are allocated;
   - The ways that roles and responsibilities in the funding of CME/CPD are assumed.

2. A workshop on CME/CPD was held on 3 December 1997 entitled '*CME and CPD for hospital doctors: expectations and responsibilities*' and a report was presented to SCOPME in March 1998. The workshop report is published in full as Annex 3 of this document.

3. An enquiry was commissioned by SCOPME about the ways in which career grade doctors and dentists in three NHS trusts in England choose, carry out and evaluate CPD and CME activities. Following a tendering process the study was carried out by Soundings Research and its report *Giving credit where credit is due* was considered by SCOPME in June 1998. A report of this enquiry is published in full as Annex 4 of this document.

The outputs from this work have been analysed by the steering group with their respective authors, and these discussions have been reported to SCOPME. This document summarises and draws conclusions from this work. It also makes recommendations about future strategies and responsibilities concerning continuing professional development, encompassing the process of continuing education for hospital doctors and dentists.

Conclusions and recommendations

A full appreciation of the many complex issues that underlie SCOPME's conclusions and recommendations requires a knowledge of the background documentation published as part of this document as well as a report earlier this year, *Doctors & Dentists: The need for a process of review*. A key recommendation in this latter report was:

> *The medical and dental professions should make a commitment that all doctors and dentists will take part in a process of review during which they would have the opportunity and be assisted to reflect and analyse their own performance, informed by the views of their peers and in the context of nationally agreed standards and local needs, and helped to take action to capitalise on their strengths and remedy any weaknesses.*

SCOPME recommended that action on this should be taken by the medical and dental professions through their leading bodies.

Based on all of this work and taking account of the recent government initiatives to promote quality in the NHS, SCOPME reiterates and expands its view on CPD as follows:

- CPD is the individual component of a collective process focused on enhancing professional and clinical effectiveness. Clinicians pursue careers within the setting of a practice community, and it is through participation in the practices of that community that careers are advanced and service innovation developed. **It is the capacity of the practice community to provide and support opportunities for innovation, experiment and change which lies at the heart of CPD;**

- CPD is a process belonging to the individual clinician that has to be complemented by a collective perspective which recognises that development of the individual is embedded in the development of the practice community;
- CPD should respond to service requirements rather than be seen to be in conflict with them;
- CPD should be linked to a general process of review,[4] at trust and directorate level, of all career grade staff which will allow regular and prospective planning of a clinician's educational needs and review of their past achievements. Such a process, which may include formal arrangements for appraisal — however this shall be defined[5] — should be given serious consideration as an alternative to current methods of validating the commitment of doctors and dentists to continuing education.

SCOPME therefore recommends that:

CPD should be much better publicised and explained to doctors and dentists within the context of the development of clinical governance and incorporating the broader concept of CPD as described by SCOPME rather than limited to a narrower debate about the future of continuing education for individual doctors and dentists.

SCOPME concludes that CPD should be developed in ways that are consistent with, and accountable to, the professional and ethical obligations that clinicians recognise as benefiting themselves and their patients and to which they are committed. Good practice in CPD should be judged not by what can be measured easily nor by what has the greatest public visibility. Rather it should be judged by the extent to which is promotes the practical expression of these professional and ethical values.

As a consequence, SCOPME considers that CME and CPD activities cannot be justified solely on the grounds that they conform to college requirements. Rather, a professional and ethical justification must be developed to give a convincing rationale for specific activities showing how they enhance and advance the service, clinical practice and patient care.

SCOPME therefore recommends that:

Doctors and dentists, having recognised CME and CPD as a professional and ethical obligation which is of direct benefit to them and their patients, should articulate rationales and justifications for, and give an account of, their CME/CPD activities in ways that indicate clearly how such activities enhance understanding and promote the development of services, clinical practice and patient care within the context of their present and future roles.

Recommendations for trust chief executives and medical directors

Trust chief executives and medical directors have a key role in promoting CPD. They will be responsible for the quality of the clinical service provided in trusts and will implement the new processes required by clinical governance. SCOPME considers that more could be done at trust level with representatives of the medical royal colleges to ensure that CME and CPD activities are better tailored to local and individual needs.

References and Notes
4.   SCOPME. *Doctors & Dentists: The need for a process of review.* 1999.
5.   SCOPME has so far only considered and defined appraisal for doctors and dentists in training (see SCOPME. *Appraising doctors and dentists in training. a working paper for consultation.* 1996).

SCOPME therefore recommends that:

NHS trusts and other health care employers, both inside and outside the NHS should:

a. Promote and support the initiatives relating to CPD in the Department of Health's consultative document, A first class service: quality in the new NHS, incorporating the broader concept of CPD as described by SCOPME;

b. Recognise CPD as a means to service development and innovation through support for, and investment in, the maintenance of quality of their medical and dental staff, and take appropriate action;

c. Recognise that CPD needs adequate and equitable funding to enable individual doctors and dentists to promote and develop their own career plans, in the context and in the interests of the teams or practice communities in which they work, and take appropriate action;

d. Recognise the effect that time constraints and other barriers have in disrupting educational participation within practice communities, and take appropriate action;

e. Work with medical royal colleges to develop an integrated approach to the organisation of CPD and peer review at a local level.

Recommendations for medical royal colleges and their faculties

Medical royal colleges have a responsibility to their members and fellows to promote CPD and CME. In the current climate of public and governmental distrust in the continuing competence of all doctors and dentists, and the perceived need for validation of specialists, the colleges have a unique opportunity to adopt and promote better methods for validating CPD and CME which should be based on the needs of the individual. SCOPME's enquiries suggest that current college CME policies are both prescriptive and limited, and concentrate too much on achieving a credit score. Such scores do not necessarily reflect a broad enough scope for self-motivated learning, and may inhibit some doctors or dentists from pursuing an educational strategy that would suit their own interests, those of practice communities in which they work and those of their employers.

SCOPME therefore recommends that:

The medical royal colleges and their faculties for the hospital specialties should:

a. Develop and publicise, on a national, regional and local basis, innovative ways to help their members and fellows comply with strategies designed to meet the needs of their own and other specialties;

b. Modify their methods of classifying and recording CPD and CME activities. There is ample scope to develop, in liaison with NHS trusts, schemes which provide opportunities for clinicians to articulate their developmental expectations and approaches, indicating the benefits derived from such activity, and describing the potential impact on services, clinical practice and patient care;

c. Develop, in liaison with NHS trusts, a system for peer review and appraisal as a potential means of assessing CPD and CME participation.

Recommendations for all stakeholders

Previous SCOPME publications have proposed general principles for CPD and have emphasised the need for greater collaboration between stakeholders in promoting professional development for doctors and dentists.

SCOPME recognises that such collaboration will require a major culture change to ensure the implementation of the CPD process. To synchronise with the development of clinical governance in NHS hospitals,

SCOPME therefore recommends that:

There is an urgent need for representatives of the stakeholders, including the doctors and dentists themselves, to develop an integrated approach to the organisation and management of CPD.

How this report is structured

The output from the workshop held in December 1997 and the enquiry in three trusts by Soundings Research are summarised in Sections 2 and 3. Section 4 contains a synthesis of the principles underlying CPD and CME drawn from the three programmes. The Annexes comprise a list of members of the steering group, membership of SCOPME, the full workshop report and the full Soundings Research report on the enquiry in three trusts.

2 Summary of a workshop on CME and CPD for hospital doctors — Expectations and responsibilities

See Annex 3, page 17 for a full report of the workshop. The views expressed are those of the workshop participants.

A workshop for invited participants was held at SCOPME on 3 December 1997. Professor Prys-Roberts introduced the workshop with a premise that:

> *'Every NHS and private sector patient has a right to expect that the doctor or dentist treating them, be they specialists or non-specialists, has been properly trained for the purpose and has maintained his or her skills and knowledge throughout their career'.*

The objective of the workshop was to resolve a perceived conflict between the provision of medical and dental services, and the needs of the professionals — doctors and dentists, consultants and other career grades — to promote and enhance their personal career objectives, while at the same time enhancing the quality of care for their patients.

Four components of the CPD/CME process were proposed as important criteria in attempting to identify the causes of conflict, and their potential resolution:

- **Opportunities:** how might the employer (the NHS trusts) optimise the enabling and funding of CPD and CME in the interests of maintaining a well-trained and updated workforce?
- **Planning:** how could doctors and dentists plan their own career development in an innovative way, rather than having it planned for them by others, for example their professional bodies? How could such plans be matched with the service requirements, present and future, of the NHS trust or other healthcare employer?
- **Delivery:** to identify better and more innovative ways of achieving CME, emphasising self-directed learning and reflective practice.
- **Outcome:** to reconcile the availability of time and funding of the individual professional's optimal learning process with the service demand and improved quality of patient care on behalf of the employer.

The conclusions of the workshop

Workshop participants gave a clear indication of some major directional changes which are required if the CPD/CME process is to become more widespread and effective.

- CPD, as a process encompassing CME, should be organised locally at NHS trust level to enable and encourage the individual doctor or dentist to develop a life-long habit of self-assessment, and self-motivated learning. The trusts have a prime responsibility to support this process because in order to provide high-quality healthcare for the patient, they must be seen to employ and maintain the highest quality medical staff. This concept is entirely consistent with the principles of 'clinical governance' which has emerged during the past year as a Government platform for the developing of the NHS as a quality service.
- CPD belongs to the individual practitioner, but NHS trusts should be encouraged to develop programmes to ensure the provision of time and adequate funding to

facilitate the process. Moreover, they should search for mechanisms to minimise disruption by service demands to participation of doctors and dentists in educational processes. The organisation of CPD/CME at trust level should reflect national and international policy for specialty development.

- Individual doctors and dentists, in consultant and non-consultant career grades, should be encouraged to develop forward-looking plans for their own CPD and CME, establishing a culture of life-long learning and maintenance of skills and knowledge. Local peer-review mechanisms for regular formal appraisal of doctors and dentists should be established to assist and validate the efforts of individual practitioners. Such appraisal should be part of the clinical governance process, and should include methods for both the validation and quantification of CME.

- Although the medical royal colleges have established a role in the quantification and validation of certain aspects of CME for their members and fellows, there was a strong perception by workshop participants that there is a need for a culture change, and a greater collaboration between the trusts and the colleges. The present 'credits system' was seen by many practitioners as being irrelevant to their existing self-education process, and frequently failed to encompass all the activities from which they could learn, including patient care, informal discussions with colleagues, reading and preparation for teaching.

- Medical royal colleges have important contributions to make in setting standards and guidelines for learning, in the continued provision of various categories of CME, and in assessing the outcome of the educational process as it affects their specialism. The colleges were also perceived to have a role in assessing the service needs of a trust with respect to the relevant specialism, and assisting their members and fellows to tailor their educational needs in the light of their everyday practice.

3 Summary of an enquiry into CME/CPD in three NHS trusts — Giving credit where credit is due

See Annex 4, page 45 for a full report of this enquiry.

An enquiry into CME/CPD in three NHS trusts was commissioned by SCOPME from Soundings Research (Bill Fleming, Lesley Golding and Pat Fleetwood-Walker) and their report was considered in June 1998. The full report is published as Annex 4 of this document.

The Soundings Research study was designed to evaluate how career grade doctors and dentists in three NHS trusts:

- Choose their CPD/CME activities;
- Perceive access to CPD/CME opportunities;
- Judge the effectiveness of what they do.

The study was qualitative and used single in-depth interviews (30–45 minutes) to question 66 professionals, across a wide range of specialisms, in a 'teaching' hospital, a district general hospital and a community trust. The total included 16 clinical directors, a director of medical education, one clinical tutor, three medical directors and a personnel officer. Thus the professionals were interviewed in both their clinical and managerial roles.

The interview material was used to derive a model of CPD/CME activity describing the key concepts in the analytical framework of the study. From the analysis of this material, the authors concluded that the role of **personal, professional and organisational identity,** within a team approach to their specialism and its service, was a key component in hospital doctors' and dentists' choice of CPD/CME activities. The combination of salient identity factors was shown to give rise to an approach to CPD/CME which clinicians used both to plan and evaluate their choices and the effectiveness of the process.

The authors also identified **'practice communities'** as important cohorts, representing a variety of formal and informal, internal and external professional groups, teams, gatherings, associations and societies; through participation in which the identity of the individual professional as a learner and knowledge seeker develops. A number of factors were identified which disrupt participation in such practice communities and therefore opportunities for service-relevant continuing learning.

On the evidence of the interview material, CPD was not a widely recognised concept, whereas CME was understood and undertaken by all those interviewed. While some exceeded levels of CME activity suggested by their royal college, a small number found difficulty in meeting college requirements. Four categories of CME activity were recognised:

- Elective CME — participation in formal opportunities;
- Routine activity — work-related meetings, including audit;
- Informal interaction with colleagues;
- Learning activity triggered by direct patient care;
- Reading was also acknowledged as an important source of learning, although mostly undertaken in clinicians' own time.

CME was described by clinicians in management positions as:

- A matter between individuals and royal colleges; but perceived in a number of ways:
  - 'Them and us' — CME system set up by colleges as a form of surveillance;
  - 'An irritation but broadly complied with';
  - 'A good thing to persuade others to pursue CME, but not necessary for me';
  - 'A framework which helps individuals to structure their learning activity';
- A joint responsibility between the trusts and the royal colleges, or
- A joint responsibility between individual professionals and their trust.

In none of the three trusts was CME/CPD managed by the trust through mechanisms such as business planning, quality, risk or human resource management. Moreover, it was characterised by variable levels of funding which were reflected in a varying culture of taking study leave.

Disruption of participation in practice communities

The study identified a number of factors which disrupted clinicians' access to, and participation in, their practice communities and thereby reduced their opportunities for service relevant continuing learning.

- Ignoring development needs arising from changing identities results in isolation of the clinician from the practice community. Some of the relevant factors are:
  - 'Geographical isolation';
  - 'Heavy service workloads';
  - 'Competition with colleagues for inadequate resources';
- Imposition of CME systems with purposes extrinsic to the core values and principles of the relevant practice community, i.e:
  - 'CME systems are not perceived as being designed to directly foster professionalism and benefit patient care;
  - 'Royal college CME points and credits systems were seen as diverting energy and resources from the core values of the professional community;
  - 'Such systems were perceived as other-directed and other-regulated, rather than fostering self-direction and self-regulation;
- Lack of resources to enable full participation:
  - 'Time is the main resource which career grade doctors and dentists need in order to participate in an appropriate range of CPD/CME activities, either within the practice community, or externally';
  - 'Time given for study leave is not equitably distributed across the career grades';
  - 'Study leave is not necessarily protected time, and such leave may not be usable because of service demands';
  - 'Funding is a necessary resource to enable participation';
  - 'CME budgets are not identified clearly';
  - 'Availability of, and access to, library and information sources vary'.
- Many staff grade and other non-consultant career grade doctors work in isolation from consultants, feel marginalised in their trust, blocked in their careers, and neglected by the royal colleges.

The Soundings Research report drew three major conclusions:

- Enhancing participation in practice communities can best be achieved by encouraging and supporting such communities as key places of learning and working to reduce and eliminate the causes of disruption to participation;

- Most doctors and dentists interviewed have developed, or are in the process of developing, a habit and culture of continuing education tailored to their individual needs. This involves engagement with a range of practice community activities. Much of this activity is central to continuing education and professional development, although it is 'invisible' to the royal colleges' CME system, e.g. reading;

- Clinicians' patterns of participation in CME have a scope, coherence and structure which, while not amounting to rational planning, is far from ad hoc. Trusts and royal colleges facilitate, but sometimes disrupt, such engagement and participation.

A synthesis of principles underlying CPD and CME drawn from this enquiry

This section elaborates some of the themes that have emerged from this project and which form the basis for the recommendations made in Section 1.

Two major themes have emerged from both the workshop and the Soundings Research report:

- The concept of CPD is not recognised widely, neither by individual doctors and dentists, nor by their employing trusts. By contrast, CME is strongly associated with royal colleges' credits and activity schemes;
- There is clear identification of the role of individual practitioners (doctors and dentists) in sustaining a self-motivated and self-directed learning process throughout their professional lives. Such a process, while reflecting a personal, moral and ethical obligation enshrined in the concept of professionalism, should also fulfil the premise of the patient's expectation.

CPD and clinical governance

At the start of the steering group's enquiries, two questions were posed:

- Is there evidence that expenditure on CPD and CME represents good value for money?
- Is there evidence of improved outcomes for patient care as a result of CPD and CME?

Although those responsible for managing resources for CME and CPD activities will no doubt still be concerned with the first of these, the second question has perhaps been overtaken by events and the value of CME and CPD appears to be no longer questioned.

Subsequent to the last meeting of the steering group, the government issued a consultation document *A first class service: quality in the new NHS*, setting out a formidable agenda for improving quality, standards, efficiency, openness and accountability. Clinical governance, defined as a framework for organisational and individual responsibility and accountability for quality in the NHS, is identified as a key process linked to professional self-regulation and life-long learning as a means to deliver improved quality.

A major item in the new agenda is continuing professional development (CPD) which is identified by the Department of Health as:

'A process of lifelong learning for all individuals and teams which meets the needs of patients and delivers the health outcomes and healthcare priorities of the NHS and which enables professionals to expand and fulfil their potential.'

In its response to the document, SCOPME suggested that a more appropriate definition would be:

'CPD is a process of lifelong learning that enables professionals to expand and fulfil their personal and professional potential and thereby meet the present and future needs of patients and deliver the health outcomes and health care priorities of the NHS.'

Implicit in the government's definition is an acceptance that CPD <u>will</u> deliver improved outcome. This is supported by a statement that:

> *'Patients and their families place their trust in health professionals. They need to be assured that their treatment is up to date and effective and is provided by those whose skills have kept pace with new thinking and new techniques.'*

Much of this reflects the broad consensus on the principles of continuing professional development for doctors and dentists, as evidenced in the recent Chief Medical Officer's report on CPD in general practice[6] and the General Dental Council's paper on recertification.[7]

Within the proposed clinical governance framework, CPD is defined clearly as a responsibility of the local health employers and, in the case of hospital doctors and dentists, the NHS trusts:

> *'In an increasingly competitive labour market, local health employers must recognise the value of appropriately managed CPD programmes in attracting, motivating and retaining high-calibre professionals...'*

and:

> *'Health professionals, professional bodies and local employers need to discuss a locally-based approach to CPD, centred on the service development needs of the community and the learning needs of the individual.'*

Thus there is ample evidence in the Department of Health's consultative document that SCOPME's previous views on CPD have informed the Department's current thinking which places the emphasis on the learning needs of the individual. However, the Soundings Research study suggests that this offers a rather one-dimensional notion of CPD which ignores the significance of the various practice communities through which CPD is made possible and is either enhanced or constrained. An overemphasis on the individual ignores the perception that clinical work and innovation in practice is realised through group or team collective activity at various levels. Keeping the service up to date and responding to development is therefore not simply centred on individuals but on the co-ordinated activity of the members of the practice community.

The role of appraisal in CPD

An important conclusion of the SCOPME workshop was that regular appraisal of the career doctor or dentist is an appropriate mechanism for the assessment and planning of the individual's professional needs, and subsequently for reviewing the implementation and outcome of those plans. Reference was made at the workshop to 'personal development portfolios' as a means of planning the life-long learning of the clinician within a team framework, and within the perceived service requirements of the trust or other employer.

The workshop considered that appraisal, in the form of a peer review process, should be organised locally. However, because they have a clearer perception of matters relevant to the specialty than do trust officers, the medical royal colleges should become involved in the development of the appraisal process. In conjunction with the postgraduate deans, the colleges have already recognised and established appraisal as a

References

6. Department of Health. *A review of continuing professional development in general practice.* A report by the Chief Medical Officer. 1998.
7. General Dental Council. *Reaccreditation and recertification for the dental profession: a document for consultation.* London: GDC, 1997.

key process for doctors and dentists in training, and that expertise should be valuable in applying the same principles to career grade doctors and dentists. To meet these new needs, the colleges might wish to develop a parallel system to that of the college 'specialty tutor' for specialist training, and to develop educational programmes in the process of peer review.

Because of the very different meanings attached to the word 'appraisal' by different groups, SCOPME has only included the term 'peer review' in its recommendations. Before 'appraisal' is adopted widely in the professions there needs to be agreement about its purpose and process.

The role of professional bodies (the medical royal colleges and specialty associations) in CPD and CME

A key emerging issue, arising from both the workshop and the Soundings Research enquiry, is that there are major tensions between the individual doctor's or dentist's objectives and their achievement, and the prescriptive processes and systems devised by the medical royal colleges as a means of quantifying and classifying the doctor's or dentist's participation. The colleges' current CME systems are seen as an inadequate instrument to ensure the initial and continuing competence of specialists.

The Soundings Research report further shows that practitioners may either:

- Completely ignore the college 'credits' system while sustaining a self-motivated and self-directed educational programme, or
- By responding slavishly to a 'credits' goal, fail to realise the objectives of such a goal and find themselves in conflict with their desire and ability to realise their own ambitions.

The report questions whether the colleges' credits system is consistent with the principle of self-directed learning, reflecting similar uncertainties expressed in the enquiry about systems for audit, appraisal and personal development planning.

Another major theme of the Soundings Research report is the perception that while the colleges' credit system has reinforced a relationship between the practitioner and their College, it may inadvertently have caused a severance of the relationship between the practitioner and the trust in relation to CPD/CME needs. Despite the limitations of the small sample of NHS trusts in the Soundings Research enquiry, it would seem that specialists and non-specialists already take part in a wide variety of self-educational exercises outwith the college guidelines, and which are largely invisible to the college 'credits system'.

This finding reinforces the need for trusts and medical royal colleges to find ways of working together on CPD. There is a need for a clear role definition; for example, the part to be played by clinical directors in CPD. This role is difficult to develop while the CME axis is predominantly between the clinician and the college; indeed it keeps the trust out of the game except as a benevolent parent providing time and resources. The new proposals for clinical governance will only change this if the trusts can be brought in as more proactive players with the colleges and their members and fellows.

The Soundings Research report confirms and enhances the information and insights gained from Dr Baughan's review of costs, and it emphasises how inadequate resources of time and/or funding can influence how, and to what extent, doctors and dentists pursue CPD and CME.

There is an urgent need for the medical royal colleges to review their role and influence on the CPD and CME processes, maximising their options for influencing the necessary culture change among their members and fellows. Together with specialty associations and societies, the royal colleges are best equipped to:

- Advise their members and fellows of their responsibilities and obligations as professionals within a specific specialty setting;

- Define the core and specialised skills and knowledge base appropriate for clinicians, both consultants and non-consultants, to keep abreast of new developments within that specialty;
- Advise trusts and other healthcare employers of these developments;
- Encourage their members and fellows to develop and maintain a self-motivated life-long learning process.

The question of non-compliance

A recurring theme in Soundings Research report is that most of the doctors and dentists questioned were actively pursuing CME, either according to their college criteria or their own. The current credits system is seen largely as a lever to deal with non-compliance with college requirements rather than a positive incentive to develop and sustain competence. There was a widespread concern that the colleges are devoting their energies to the compliant majority as a means of coercing the reluctant minority. However, these clinicians also recognise that a small proportion of their colleagues, often described as 'laggards', fail to keep up to date and maintain their clinical standards.

Given the new emphasis by government and the General Medical Council on clinical performance rather than on achieving educational credits, SCOPME considers that trust chief executives, the medical royal colleges, the General Medical Council and the government need to collaborate in the development of more meaningful arrangements for ensuring that doctors can and do keep up to date and achieve local and national requirements. Such systems should remain distinct from, but should also complement, arrangements for CPD which are designed to enhance the personal, professional and organisational abilities of doctors and dentists within their present roles in practice communities and in the longer term.

A1 | Members of the SCOPME CPD steering group

Professor Cedric Prys-Roberts (chair), SCOPME member
Mr Graham Elderfield, Chief Executive, Isle of Wight Healthcare NHS Trust
Dr David Percy, Director of Postgraduate General Practice Education, NHSE South West
Professor Colin Coles, SCOPME member
Ms Jane McCue, Clinical Director of Surgery, East Hertfordshire NHS Trust
Mr Malcolm Pendlebury, Dean, Faculty of General Dental Practitioners (UK)
Dr Jammi Rao, Consultant in Public Health Medicine, Sandwell Health Authority
Dr Peter Wilkinson, SCOPME member
Dr Annabelle Baughan (Project Director)
Mr David O'Carroll (Observer, NHSE)

SCOPME Membership

(Immediately prior to its disbandment on 31 March 1999)

Professor Dame Barbara Clayton, Hon. research professor in metabolism, Southampton University (chairman)
Dr Trevor Bayley, Postgraduate dean, North West region, Mersey deanery, Liverpool (vice-chairman)
Professor Robert Boyd, Principal, St George's Hospital Medical School, London
Dame Fiona Caldicott, Principal, Somerville College, Oxford
Professor Colin Coles, Institute of Health and Community Studies, Bournemouth University
Miss Constance Fozzard, Consultant obstetrician and gynaecologist, Truro, Cornwall
Professor John Frame, Postgraduate dental dean, West Midlands region, Birmingham
Dr Steve Hajioff, Specialist Registrar in Public Health Medicine, South Essex Heath Authority, Brentwood, Essex
Mr Bryan Harrison, Chief Executive, Forest Healthcare Trust, Essex
Mrs Celia Ingham Clark, Consultant surgeon, Whittington Hospital, London
Dr Eddie Josse, General practitioner, London
Mrs Rita Lewis, Health policy consultant, Coulsdon, Surrey
Professor Cedric Prys-Roberts, Professor of anaesthetics, University of Bristol
Dr Sam Ramaiah, Director of public health medicine, Walsall Health Authority
Mr Stephen Rear, General dental practitioner, Henley-on-Thames
Dr Deborah Richardson-Kelly, Associate regional postgraduate dean (human resources) and hon. consultant in public health medicine (medical manpower), North East and Yorkshire region, Newcastle upon Tyne
Mr David Rule, Postgraduate dental dean, Thames regions, Thames Postgraduate Medical and Dental Education, London
Dr Peter Wilkinson, Consultant physician, Ashford Hospital NHS Trust, Middlesex

Assessors
For the General Medical Council:
Professor Charles George, Dean, Faculty of Medicine, Health and Biological Sciences, Southampton University

For the General Dental Council:
Mr Trevor Griffiths, General dental practitioner, Cardigan, Dyfed

Observers:
Dr Graham Buckley, Executive director, Scottish Council for Postgraduate and Continuing Medical and Dental Education, Edinburgh
Professor Tom Hayes, Postgraduate dean and secretary, Welsh Council for Postgraduate Medical Education, Cardiff
Dr Jack McCluggage, Postgraduate dean and chief executive, Northern Ireland Council for Postgraduate Medical Education, Belfast
Mr Robin Naysmith, Head of Medical Education Unit, NHSE Headquarters, Leeds

CME and CPD for hospital doctors: expectations and responsibilities

A report of a SCOPME workshop held on 3 December 1997

Introduction

In his introduction, the workshop chairman, Professor Cedric Prys-Roberts said that every NHS and private sector patient had a right to expect that every specialist or non-specialist treating them had been properly trained and has maintained his or her skills and knowledge throughout their career. There is a clear conflict between the demands of providing a service and the needs of the professionals to promote and enhance their career objectives, while at the same time enhancing the quality of care for the patients.

This workshop was aimed at addressing this dichotomy, to listen to varied viewpoints and to define participants' expectations and perceived responsibilities, and, hopefully, to arrive at a consensus. In designing the workshop the SCOPME steering group had accepted the validity of the premise that CPD, and its major component CME, are worthwhile objectives. The workshop concentrated therefore on four components of the process. By the end of the workshop it was hoped to have decided the priorities to be given to each of these processes, and possibly have identified more worthwhile objectives.

Components of CME/CPD

Professor Prys-Roberts identified the following components:

1. **Opportunities:** how these can be maximised through the funding and enabling of CPD and CME, based on the premise that it is in the interests of the employer to maintain a well trained and updated workforce.

2. **Planning:** using innovative ways through which doctors and dentists can plan their own professional development and continuing education rather than having it planned for them by others, for instance, by the professional bodies. How can individuals match their plans with the opportunities provided for them by their employer?

3. **Delivery (particularly of CME):** we need to identify better and more innovative ways of delivering CME. We need to consider aspects such as self-directed learning and reflective practice, including the facilitation of education in small groups for individuals who do not have the opportunity to work in a large learning environment. Learning portfolios need to be considered together with ways in which they can be used as a rigorous method for capturing evidence of reflective practice, as a potentially useful means of assessing and accrediting CME, rather than the 'brownie points' system existing at present. Distance learning packages also need to be considered.

4. **Outcome:** this should be considered not only in terms of improvements in patient care, important though that is. At the same time the aspect of job satisfaction should not be overlooked and also satisfaction for the purchasers and providers of CME. In the summary of their report to the Chief Medical Officer on the effectiveness of CPD, Stanton and Grant state that their review of the literature has shown no educational panacea, no most effective learning method, no 'best buy' outcome measures. They also state that the effectiveness of CPD is a function of the process. We must focus on improving the quality of that process and making it more relevant to individual needs, service needs, the needs of the team or the practice.

INVITED PRESENTATIONS: EXPECTATIONS AND RESPONSIBILITIES

The viewpoint of the individual doctor
Dr Peter Wilkinson — consultant cardiologist at Ashford Hospital, Middlesex and Harefield Hospital and a member of SCOPME

I work at a small district general hospital and also in a specialist centre which provides me with the opportunity to interact with other specialists. This particular outside link helps me enormously. Box 1 lists the self-evident responsibilities of the individual doctor.

Box 1: The responsibilities of the individual doctor

- Maintenance of knowledge, skills and attitudes
- Keeping up to date with relevant advances
- Inclusion of broader CPD curriculum
- Awareness of educational needs
- Inclusion of community and institutional needs
- Risk management topics

An example of the maintenance of knowledge and skills which I have experienced personally is having to re-learn the skills of permanent pacing when this was introduced into my DGH from the tertiary centre. From past experience it is not always the case that training and maintenance of skills accompany new techniques, e.g. minimally invasive surgery. It is important for me to keep up to date with relevant advances in general medicine and in my specialty, but also to be abreast of the broader CPD curriculum and not just the narrow CME focus. This includes communications and appraisal skills and management techniques. Awareness of educational needs is important. Many doctors indulge in a very hit and miss approach to their CME and CPD with no consideration of the longer term planning process to match the needs of the workplace — of the department, of the hospital — and there needs to be a process of incorporating those needs in personal educational plans. Risk management topics also need to be considered from an educational viewpoint.

There needs to be the right balance in the methods of learning, for example journal reading, external conferences. Research in Canada by Dr Davis showed that some approaches are more effective than others and he listed four approaches which he noted were used very effectively by pharmaceutical companies. Drug companies are skilled in creating change in doctors, using opinion leaders, outreach visits and multifaceted activities, and we should learn from that. Davis in his review article points out that audit, even with feedback, is less effective that this multifaceted approach. Formal CME conferences without other strategies have relatively little impact. We need therefore to examine the educational activities to ensure the quality of educational experiences is a good one. There needs to be active involvement in internal and external CME and not just because the Royal College requires participation. A balanced approach to the time spent on CME is important. It is not possible to read all of the medical journals and therefore we need to manage what we need to know.

Not all CME costs money but invariably there are opportunity costs in terms of not being available to see patients. Employers do provide paid study leave but this is very often insufficient. As a profession we have an obligation to fund some of that leave personally. After attending CME lectures there is also an obligation to spread the word among colleagues by telling them about what you've learned.

At the institutional level doctors should be moving towards a regular system of reflecting with another practitioner and negotiating a programme for a period of 12-months ahead. This could be done as part of a job plan or personal appraisal. The doctor should expect some time and funding for this from the employer. The role of the chief executive of supporting a learning organisation is crucial. Doctors are more privileged than other staff, such as nurses, in terms of access to CME/CPD. It is important that all members of the team are able to participate in CPD and doctors should support this.

The expectations of commissioners should include an insistence that employers (trusts) include educational programmes in their contracts. Funding would need to be provided within contracts for CME for all staff.

Colleges and faculties should move away from counting points and encourage the process of moving towards negotiated CME/CPD personal plans for consultants. They should provide a resource of available courses as the information about availability is often not very clear. Information technology such as the Internet could be utilised far more by course providers than is currently the case. Colleges need to encourage CME and educational programmes that make a change.

In conclusion:
- Much of doctors' CME is *ad hoc*;
- Counting CME points/hours has not made much difference.

The view of patients
Mr (now Lord) Toby Harris, Director of the Association of Community Health Councils, England and Wales.

Everyone has been a patient but we all get treated differently. I was speaking at a conference somewhere in central London and during the course of the morning I began to feel increasingly ill. I then found myself some time later in my local accident and emergency department. The first thing they do to you as a patient is they take away your clothes. It is very difficult to be an articulate and forthright patient when they have taken away your clothes. In my case they had given me a gown which did not fit terribly well. So I did not feel at my most effective when this young house doctor picked up the notes and asked me as they are trained to do 'Tell me Mr Harris', and this was after he had asked me how much I drank 'What do you do for a living?' Now of course what I should have done at this stage is lied if I really wanted to know how the health service in that particular hospital treats patients. But I said 'I am the Director of the Association of Community Health Councils'. A brief pause while I explained to him what a Community Health Council was. And then he went round the back of the curtain and I could hear him phoning the registrar and he said 'I really do think you should come down. Well he says he is the Director of the Association of Community Health Councils'.

My reason for telling that story is that I suspect for very many professionals it is extremely difficult to know what it is like to be a patient receiving the treatment that you give. When you are a senior professional, when you are a senior manager, somehow when you arrive at the Outpatients Department or at the Accident & Emergency Department or are booked in for a planned admission, the word goes round and you are not treated in quite the same way as you might be if you were the normal patient off the street or the ambulance.

An expectation that patients should have of the whole CME and CPD process is about making sure that an understanding of being a patient is incorporated into the learning. We should see to it that there is a significant role for patients or patients' representatives in drawing up the curriculum, the content of large amounts of CME and CPD. There is also considerable scope for direct participation by users of the service in teaching what it feels like and what it really is like to be a patient.

The basic expectation for patients is that they need to be assured that professionals are up-to-date. They need to feel that the person they go and see does know what is going on; that they are aware, in broad terms but not in every detail, of all that is going on in the medical journals. And this is going to become an increasing expectation and an increasing requirement. You will increasingly find that patients arrive having already virtually diagnosed themselves and decided what treatment is now the leading edge that they ought to be demanding. First of all it will be necessary not to have a sort of blank look and say 'I've never heard of that' and it will be necessary to be able to explain to the patient why that particular treatment or that particular diagnosis may not in fact be the most appropriate in their particular case. And it is going to require a much greater sharing of information, and the only way that the professional is going to be able do that is by themselves being up-to-date and aware of the sorts of debates and discussions that are going on elsewhere.

We would also argue that the content of CME should reflect that professionals should be aware of patients' rights and of sources of advice and information for patients. While I think there will be many patients who will increasingly, with the information explosion, turn up extremely well informed and well advised, I think there will always remain those who will not know their way around information sources, or how to find their way to where they can get advice, or know their rights. So they need to be guided through them.

This is part of ensuring that CME and CPD does not just focus on clinical developments, but focuses on the on-going cultural change in health services. In the future professionals are going to be fulfilling a role, perhaps much more than they have in the past, which is about facilitating patient choice, enabling patients to be full partners in both treatment decisions and in the care that they receive. And that is going to require not only the communications skills which I mentioned earlier, but it is also going to require an understanding and an acceptance of that change in culture. Now that is something that is already happening increasingly in medical schools but I think it is something that needs to be passed on and reflected in CME and CPD.

There remains a worry for many patients that professionals are exposed to too much new thinking, and that there may be some professionals who are itching to use new techniques or to try something out that they have read about to see whether it is quite as exciting as everyone says. And so the other expectation from patients is that there is adequate training before professionals let themselves loose on new techniques and new ideas, and that we need to be sure that continuing medical education does not encourage people to try things when they have not had adequate training or experience to use them. There is an interesting balance which needs to be struck in working out how to do this. You want continuing education to enable people to move into new areas and to embrace new techniques but it needs to provide sufficient and adequate training so that people are not encouraged to do it when they are not yet ready to do so.

The experience and expertise that many patients would bring suggests that you need to use different forms of learning, different ways of getting the message across. And we are particularly interested in making sure that it is seen as equally valid to participate in clinical audit and peer review processes, and be involved in patient feedback as part of this process of continuing professional development as reading complicated research reports and attending lectures.

Finally, two points about the direction in which some of this may go. First, we are very conscious, as a patients' organisation, that the debate on rationing is slowly changing into a debate about effectiveness. Rather than politicians wanting to make difficult choices about whether certain things will or will not be affordable on the health service, they are now suggesting that the professionals make the decisions on whether or not particular processes are effective. There is a nagging concern at the back of our minds that CME and CPD must be about facilitating rather than restricting clinical freedom. And therefore it is important that this process is not one which is simply about telling people this treatment or this process is no longer regarded as effective, without really enabling people to make the choices that only they as clinicians can do on the basis of proper information and proper knowledge.

The second point is that we do not want doctors to attend educational events simply to have the boxes ticked and to get the necessary hours totted up. If CME and CPD are to be of any value at all, people who attend have to be participating fully. We have to look at ways in which you can assess the extent to which people are participating, for there to be sanctions for those who are not prepared to keep themselves abreast of developments and the extent to which participation may reveal serious inadequacies in particular professionals. Then we need to look at what steps come into force to ensure that those individuals are supported by additional training or receive additional help to make sure that their professional skills are brought up to an appropriate level. And if that proves not to be possible then mechanisms have to be implemented through the General Medical Council to make sure that in the long term these clinicians are not practising as far as patients are concerned.

Things are changing very rapidly. Professionals need to embrace these changes and patients expect them to do so, but the changes are not simply about techniques and new discoveries; they are also about culture and the way in which professionals relate to patients.

The view of employers
Mrs Val Martin, Chief Executive, Lewisham NHS Trust

This is an important topic but I am not speaking on behalf of any employers' group but rather as a trust chief executive from an inner London acute general hospital which is trying to keep its service and training and research going in very difficult circumstances. I make no apologies about concentrating on CME and only touching on CPD. That is partly because I do not believe that the battle is won on CME and I actually think it is more difficult to get CME right in the field than perhaps people in higher places might realise.

My first point is that I do not actually believe that most trusts, and certainly not most chief executives, have a strong view on this subject at all. This is not due to hostility; it might occasionally be indifference because many chief executives have much more pressing issues on their plate — configuration, service reductions, budget cuts, elective reductions in the last year, trolley waits, etc. They do not know after all whether or not CME is even effective but they do have a very clear instinct that it is going to be costly if they pay attention to it. They believe that if they allow their doctors to take CME seriously they are going to be distracted from keeping the service going. And anyway there is this great tranche of people called the medical educational fraternity who will sort it out.

So an important message is that you need to get this issue much higher up on the chief executives' agenda. It matters for five reasons:

1. In the next decade hospitals will increasingly differentiate themselves into those who are leaders of the pack and those who become 'also rans'. And you cannot run an organisation without taking an interest in the quality of your core business, the clinical service, and how it is delivered, how it is provided and the clinical teams that are providing it. So it is in the interest of your organisation that if you want it to keep abreast, then you take an interest in CME.
2. Continuing education is part of an international trend. Everything is increasingly going to be about more explicit processes for checking quality, accreditation, and that practitioners are up to date. Therefore one should capitalise on the inevitable rather than be caught out by the inevitable.

3. If commissioners are worth their money they should be expecting CME as a requirement of any hospital. They should ask if the quality of care being provided in their local hospitals is being provided by doctors who are clinically up to speed, however you define that.
4. We have shortages of critical groups of staff. What will attract people to come and what will attract them to stay? The organisations that take CPD, CME and study leave seriously, or those that do not? If you do not get ahead of the game you will not recruit or retain those staff. The issue of clinical staff morale and manpower is the most critical issue facing hospitals in the next 5-10 years.
5. Lastly, CME is important for simple defensive reasons such as a clinical risk strategy. We have rising expenditure on litigation so there needs to be a process to enable a trust to be sure that its practitioners are appropriately equipped to undertake their jobs.

CME matters and trusts need to take it more seriously and chief executives need to take a personal interest. It is not solely down to the postgraduate dean's office or the clinical tutor, or the medical director to encourage. It must come from the management side as well.

My second point is that I see a great discrepancy between the ideal and the aspirations for CME and the reality on the ground. The ideal would be that we had properly organised CME and CPD for all the medical staff in my institution and for the other groups of staff as well. There would be good internal programmes as well as fully funded arrangements for allowing people access to external programmes and sufficient funding and staff to cover the work when people are elsewhere refreshing skills or learning new ones. There would be much interest from the organisation in supporting it, with enthusiasm from the individual and his or her department, clinical director and trust, and there would be plenty of time to undertake these programmes. The issue of time is the one that worries me most. The reality is that some people are enthusiastic but there are those who are not terribly interested, and that extends to trust boards as well as clinical staff.

There is insufficient cover for those who want to take CME/CPD seriously, and insufficient money to subsidise not only the cost of the programmes but also the locum cover, so that people do not feel guilty about attending the programmes. There are also clear discrepancies between what is potentially available for doctors and for other staff and that creates tension within a hospital. There is also a discrepancy between different specialties. The more specialised doctors may need to go to international conferences and this can create tensions and difficulties back at the trust. There are also practical issues about part-timers, who have to keep their skills up in just the same way as all the others but they do so in the trust's time and at the trust's expense, and are disproportionately more costly than full-timers.

Therefore I see a tremendous gap between the ideal and the reality. What do I think would help? First, funding. Currently CME is partly funded by people paying for it themselves, partly departmental soft monies, partly by some trusts contributing funds. It will not be easy for trusts to provide this money. For the last two years I could only make available £500 each for medical staff CME at a time when I have been closing beds and cancelling elective surgery. It is a real problem to find resources for CME. You probably need to allow £2,500 per consultant to cover expenses for courses and activities, and to do so seriously you would need to allow a similar amount to cover costs of absence. A minimum for trusts would be £5000 per consultant. This would mean nearly £0.5 million on my trust's bill. Across the country this could be £200–300 million. If CME is to be taken seriously, there are real costs. I see no reason why full-time practitioners working in a DGH should be paying for this mainly out of their own pocket. If they do, then this organisation and others should press the Department that at least this should be allowable for tax relief. That would be one of my practical suggestions. More importantly, this organisation should be saying to the Department that it could cost £200–300 million to put CME on a proper footing and arguably it should be ring-fenced so that it does not get diverted.

Third, we need to be more focused about what we want to achieve through CME/CPD. If we argue for more explicit public funding then we will have to expect a much more rigorous process of accountability. What does the trust get out of it? How does it improve patient care? How does a doctor's individual programme relate to the trust's overall needs? If we get real about the money we must get real about the focus. CME will need to be more formal and more explicit. It will require an organisation focus within each trust, not just CME committees and guidelines but also the medical director, clinical tutor and trust board being more serious about putting CME firmly within mainstream activities. In my trust we have an academic director and academic board as well as clinical tutor and college tutors to make sure that the whole emphasis of the organisation on training and CPD are brought into the mainstream. I would see in a year or two CME and CPD appearing in directorate business plans as they need to be allowed for and accounted for in our budgets, alongside clinical service activity. I would also expect other bodies, such as colleges, to start publishing 'white lists' and making them open and available to the public. As a trust director I would like that information. I see it all becoming much more mandatory and in the public arena, and rightly so in ethical terms, partly because of public funding and partly because up to 50 per cent of all medical knowledge becomes out of date in three or four years, compared with 10 or 15 years ago. I would wish to think that doctors and dentists in my hospital are up to date.

Lastly, I will comment on 'people issues'. As chief executive, first, how can I be fair to the other staff in my organisation in the same way I would like to be fair to the medical staff? That is a real issue. I might have 80–90 consultants but I have 2500 staff in total. If I am to give them the same time, support and resourcing, this is a major organisational issue. Sometimes when chief executives do not want to get involved with CME it is because they will then have to struggle with the more explicit question of what do we do for the other staff. Second, the medical profession as a whole needs to help chief executives to handle the issue of those who are not enthusiasts either because of workload or lack of interest. I do not want it to become a disciplinary matter between the chief executive and a member of the consultant body. I want some working arrangement built up around what is good practice, reinforced from the colleges, etc., so that it is very much seen as an expectation of the medical profession and it is not left to an individual manager to deal alone with the doctor who is not keeping up to date.

Finally, I would like the thrust to be about supporting and nurturing people and not about policing. I do not care for the words 'performance management'. It is about developing people. Estate agents selling houses think about location, location, location. The issue with CME/CPD is time, time, time. I have many committed consultants who would love to do all these programmes and to find out what they should be doing, but they are struggling with time. Expectations of them now are very great — to supervise their juniors, to do audit and research, to keep the service going, and now to do CME. I recognise that the workload and expectations we are throwing on individual doctors will cause two things to happen. Many doctors in their fifties will want to leave the profession, and many others will go for those trusts and hospitals where services are organised in much bigger clinical teams so they will get more of a breathing space in a larger set-up. Part of the challenge for us as managers is to consider how to enable them to function in a way that keeps their professional interests alive and to recognise that nobody who becomes a specialist at the age of just over 30 can be expected to stay fresh and passionate about their subject for 30 years without our creating some time and space for them.

The view of healthcare commissioners
Dr Michael Gill, Director of Public Health and Health Policy, Brent and Harrow Health Authority

First, I would like to offer a critique of the levers at the disposal of the health authority when it comes to CME and CPD. Second, I want to share with you a few thoughts on the personal and organisational development, and what implications it might have for the content and structure of CME. Third, I want you to suspend disbelief for a few minutes and imagine a few ideal types, an ideal clutch of colleges, an ideal clutch of health authorities and an ideal clutch of doctors in receipt of CME. Finally, I want to conclude by drawing attention to some of the big themes.

Levers

I am not the only person who would view what is described as contracting as little more than a remote bureaucratic process of budgetary allocation. Almost on no occasion has it even gone as far as identifying CME needs within an organisation, let alone devising ways of trying to meet them. And this is, to some extent, true of clinical audit which remains at least from the point of view of most consultants within the NHS, a largely marginal activity sustained by audit facilitators or nurses or by junior hospital doctors, with a focus primarily on in-patient process.

Workforce planning and commissioning education and training should of course be different sides of the same coin and perceived as complementary. At the moment the education consortia are a lever for what is potentially very exciting but remain inchoate. The focus of the education consortia is on workforce planning and not on the educational needs of the staff groups. This will change very quickly and the liaison between non-medical education and training and medical education and training will become greater and greater. The axis around which the postgraduate deans and health authorities revolve often amounts to last minute agreements grudgingly made or absolute flat refusals on the part of the health authority to the request for yet more junior hospital staff in a particular area, or a consultant, in an already cash-strapped trust or cash-strapped health authority. That is no way to conduct a productive relationship.

As a Director of Public Health (DPH) and a representative of the health authority, I consider the relationship with the medical director is absolutely fundamental and potentially very exciting, but has yet to realise its potential. There are many important strategic questions that arise in conversations that I have with medical directors, e.g. 'why do you want another cardiologist instead of a palliative care consultant?' If that relationship works well it allows for a very productive discussion about what steps and managerial frameworks are in place for detecting the performance of individual doctors about whom the medical director may be worried, and what role clinical directors play in developing the framework in which individuals are identified and also assisted.

Capital planning is an extremely tenuous hook on which to hang any kind of influence on CME. But occasionally there are some striking examples of a brand new way of delivering healthcare which inevitably has organisational development implications and therefore professional development implications.

Collaboration on health service research issues is almost serendipitous. But clearly if a health authority joins forces with a trust in trying to evaluate a service provided within that trust or across trusts, then whether or not the stated aims of that piece of research are met are important. The activity often shows up organisational development and professional development needs that can be dealt with. It is very tenuous in terms of the direct leverage.

General practitioners

Regarding GPs, a DPH is in the position of a medical director, but with some crucial differences. There is a very dispersed system of care delivery provided by doctors who have independent contractor status and with an extremely dispersed system of gathering intelligence about how good or bad the service is. Limited as the levers are, and in conjunction with the Local Medical Committees, we have used General Medical Services' funds, the postgraduate education allowance and medical audit advisory groups (MAAGs) to support practices where there is a real problem. The way in which MAAGs have acted as a professional development vehicle in a non-threatening fashion is something about which trusts might take note. Primary Care Act pilots and commissioning pilots provide many new opportunities for us to consider what the educational needs of the primary care teams might be.

It is obvious that professional development is part of a triad and is not to be treated in isolation. The real challenge facing what is narrowly defined as CME is how both to retain and improve doctors' technical excellence and to enable them to thrive in a multidisciplinary environment. Many doctors have a model of power and authority that is hierarchical. Much of that model has been entrenched throughout the whole of the undergraduate and, to a large extent, their postgraduate career. The whole business of learning how to express leadership in a multidisciplinary environment remains very under-explored. Yet we know that most clinical care is being delivered via teams and that the care will not be effective unless the team is itself effective; and the team will not be effective if one of its potential leaders can only think of one way of leading it. Here are three examples of where exciting progress has been made:

1. The first is in psychiatry. There are many psychiatrists who are members of a multidisciplinary team — an equal member with all the others. But they still have bottom line responsibilities when it comes to the Mental Health Act. The good ones have learnt this different way of providing influence and leadership.

2. The second example comes from outside medicine and is an example of the importance of linking professional and organisational development. Directors of finance within the NHS 10 years ago saw their role as functionaries, full of professional competence of a very narrowly defined sort to make the books balance. I would hazard a slightly provocative guess that this remains the case in a significant number of trusts. It does in some health authorities. But the good directors of finance have said 'the role is about much more than that, it's about thinking about investment for health gain not just about balancing the books'. In other words thinking about it from a public health point of view. They feel secure enough about what they do to think about their organisational role more broadly and almost leave their 'tribe'.

3. The third example is medical directors. At a conference 10 days ago for medical directors and directors of public health, I was very struck by the wide spectrum of world views represented by medical directors. At one end they understand fully how to make the most of their organisational roles and responsibilities but at the other 'thumping the tub of their tribe'.

The trouble is that most CME enhances and underpins this tribalisation because it occurs within the fold of sub-specialisation. The ideal world might be represented by a three-legged stool involving colleges, doctors and health authorities. The issue of time has been brought up on several occasions and health authorities have a responsibility via the management of the trust to negotiate time for doctors to be professional. Being professional is not just about doing CME, it is about being professional to patients as well. This is a theme that the GMC has often emphasised. But in return we will want doctors to be much more up front about what count as clinical standards. The colleges need to re-define what counts as professional. It is not just being technically competent. It is not just about knowing how to do something. Not even just about knowing what to do or when to do it — the effectiveness and the appropriateness and judgement issue — but it is also about enabling others within a team to do what they can do really well together. The whole business of what counts as good care, and how it will be expressed through the phenomenon of team-based standards, is something on which the colleges and the doctors together need to take a very strong lead.

We need to take account of the discussions that health authorities have had with their local providers over the last decade, particularly in the last five years, particularly in the last year, about what counts as a sensible catchment population for a hospital and the major strategic issues that health authorities present trusts with. But we also need to take account of the potential coalescence between some of the arguments presented by the health authorities and the lessons from Confidential Enquiry into Perioperative Deaths and other professional activities for some years, but which have been extremely difficult to embed within everyday practice. The colleges and the health authorities need to think much more about what constitutes a really good service and not run the relationship only on the basis of statements from the college saying 'this specialty needs x consultants per thousand population'. You can base a productive discussion on that kind of statement but we need to understand the arguments and everybody needs to understand the implications. The other issue is that if the imminent White Paper focuses on quality in the same way the current trust obligations focus on finance, then there is obviously a basis for a very productive two-way relationship there.

The big themes
What then are the big themes? I have used the word 'tribe' several times and this is at the heart of it. We need to be very careful that CME does not tribalise. Multidisciplinary working, people feeling comfortable in multidisciplinary teams, is going to be at the heart of success in the future and it may be at the heart of success of the profession in being able to remain self-regulatory.

'Detrustification' is a rather horrid word. If trusts are thought of as being historical accidents, reflecting the arrangements that were around in the first few years of this decade, it could be argued that designation of cancer units, for example, is essentially a feature of the existence of trusts, rather than a service based reality. In other words there are parts of cancer care which quite clearly ride right across organisational and professional boundaries, and the fact that people work within trusts may not help. Large imposed structures may not help thinking laterally within CME programmes. The same goes for thinking about vertical links. The title of today's workshop contains the words 'hospital doctors' but it may be that we will conceive of a hospital in future in a way that is not about the institution with walls. And we do need to think hard about what the implications of information technology, particularly the Internet, really will be.

Finally, we now have increasing numbers of ways of accessing health care — some of the different ways of running out-of-hours care by GPs are good recent examples. It is not always a doctor that patients need to see as a first port of call; it can be other people, nurse practitioners for example. The situation is similar in A&E. We need to regard these as opportunities not threats. And CME surely should provide us with an opportunity to develop, refine and extend our thinking on these kinds of issues. Are we sure, in thinking that we have no time to do CME, it is not because we are still doing things as a profession that others could do?

The view of the Royal Colleges
Dr Peter Toghill, Director of Continuing Medical Education, Royal College of Physicians

It is only four or five years since the colleges first promoted the concept of formal CME systems. But why is there a need for a formal system? This need seemed to emerge in the late 1980s when there were a series of medical disasters and there were public, media and political pressures on the medical profession to amend its training procedures and to review the ways in which doctors kept up to date. And at the same time, within the profession itself, there was a growing awareness of the difficulty in keeping up with the explosion of knowledge and also in finding time to get away to study. At that time there were calls for reaccreditation and re-examination. 'Why couldn't you be like the airline pilots?', everyone always used to ask. But to re-examine all the consultants in this country every five years or so would be enormously difficult. The answer seemed to be to introduce a formal system of CME that was the responsibility of the colleges.

Basically colleges had four main tasks to undertake. The first was to decide on a common strategy for CME. The second was to monitor those consultants who were taking part and to measure their activities. The third was to supervise the delivery of education and the fourth, undoubtedly the most difficult of all, to try to assess the efficacy and outcome of the whole system. Most of the colleges have similar schemes which feature:

- CME as a professional obligation;
- A target number of 50 hours per year;
- A mix of internal and external CME;
- Balanced programmes for individual doctors;
- A five-year cycle and at the end of that five years certificates of participation with perhaps a register of participation. This is the so-called 'white list' about which there has been a deal of publicity recently.

There were problems initially and it was perhaps a mistake for the individual colleges to set up their own schemes. As a result colleges started at different times, with different programmes, with different sanctions. It really needed the directors of college CME to harmonise the programmes as best they could. Things are now much better but there are still discrepancies between the colleges.

What do doctors expect from CME? From the physician's point of view, Box 4 shows how doctors rank various educational opportunities. This information is reproduced from a paper in the Journal of the Royal College of Physicians published last year. It summarises the results of a survey which showed that the most popular CME activity was reading journals. And then in decreasing order were:

- Going to meetings nationally or abroad;
- In-hospital activities;
- Informal contacts including corridor and lunchtime consultations.

and less popular:

- Reading textbooks;
- Distance learning;
- Audit (not a popular occupation).

Now that the colleges have two or three years' experience of what doctors actually do, we find that it matches up very well to this. They like going to meetings at home and away. They undertake much in-hospital education. They do not read textbooks very much. Distance learning is not very popular at the moment but perhaps this is because of its poor availability. Audit is off the bottom end of the scale. Doctors do not like audit very much — at least that is what they tell us.

I can now be devil's advocate, and suggest what I think is wrong with the college programmes. Seventy to 80 per cent of our doctors are participating in the schemes, but disappointingly they concentrate on passive lecture-format education. Cynics would say this is no more than sitting in the back row gazing at the ceiling. Currently we focus on teaching and not learning. Why do we call our hospitals 'teaching hospitals'? They should be learning hospitals! Doctors are using techniques which are known to be ineffective ways of educating professionals.

Currently we monitor attendance. We add it up in hours rather than in involvement and we do not measure the quality of our activities. Our programmes are difficult to audit and they can be expensive. What we have to remember is that adult learners have to be considered in different ways from medical students or university students. Adult learners or professionals have three major requirements. First of all, they need to look for solutions for their own specific and recognised problems. Second, they want to be involved in their own learning, and third, they are busy people and there are many demands on their time.

How can we in the colleges help doctors to recognise their own problems? We are all aware of holes in our knowledge and technology is moving so fast that it is extremely difficult to keep up. Fortunately there are now self-assessment programmes coming on stream. MCQs are being produced by the colleges and the journals; for example the Royal College of Pathologists has produced excellent MCQs to allow consultants to see how their knowledge matches with that of their peers. And I am sure you will all have seen these exciting interactive electronic packages which are now flooding on to the market. In addition we have peer review and formal audit.

Second, doctors need to be involved in their own learning and we are very fortunate in medicine in that there is much hands-on practice, and some of the colleges are introducing laboratories for skills learning. Perhaps the best example of this is the skills learning laboratory that has been developed at the Royal College of Surgeons.

Third, there are demands on time. We have heard about this today and the colleges are suggesting solutions. Obviously it is much better if there can be hospital-based meetings, and we certainly need to develop distance learning with videos and CD-Roms.

Where should the colleges go from here? We should perhaps not abandon entirely the traditional methods of lecture format meetings but graft on to these self-assessment programmes. Peer review is an extremely important and valuable method of undertaking CME, and I am very enthusiastic about learning visits, involving doctors going to see colleagues who are experts in their own field, or visiting centres of excellence. This is a much-neglected educational resource in the National Health Service. We also need to give some thought to sabbaticals. Very few NHS doctors are allowed to go on sabbaticals but I believe we should encourage this.

At the end of the day we have to try to assess competence, and this is an extremely difficult topic. We have to put together a jigsaw of factors. These include:

- A knowledge base;
- Personal skills;
- Personal log books;
- Self- and peer assessment;
- Feedback on performance;
- Ability to work in teams. No-one now works as an individual and it is critical that we all learn to work with our colleagues from within the profession and from outside the profession.

I would like to mention the 'white lists'. The Royal College of Obstetricians and Gynaecologists is unique among the colleges in that it has a mandatory CME scheme and it intends to publish its list of doctors who have completed their CME satisfactorily. How widely they are going to publish this is not known. Among the other colleges there is discussion as to what should be done with these so-called 'white lists'. No one has talked about publishing a 'blacklist' but it is not too difficult to work out who is on the 'blacklist' if you have a 'whitelist'. This is an area that perhaps is ripe for discussion and whether the publication of a 'whitelist' might be regarded as a solution.

We are three or four years along the road with formal CME. Does it make any difference? People used to ask 'Why do we need formal CME, we always did it anyhow?' I would like to pose the question '*Did* we always do it?' Many colleagues in the last 10 years of their careers tended to drift and certainly did not keep up to date. At least now CME is a professional obligation. In the past, consultants certainly kept up to date on their specialist professional knowledge. There was no problem with that. They went to their specialist meetings regularly. But they did not necessarily look at the wider aspects of medicine and in particular there was little CPD, those aspects of medicine such as management, finance, ethics, all those other professional activities which we, as colleges, are hoping to embrace within our CME schemes. In the past, much was driven by professional pride alone but I do believe that there is now an educational culture in hospitals which is growing as a result of the formal CME programmes.

A major problem that affects us all is shortage of time. When I sit in my garden I sometimes feel like saying 'Dear Lord, please just give me a little time to sit and think'.

The view of the General Medical Council
Professor Charles George, Chair of the Education Committee, General Medical Council

Under its last two presidents, the General Medical Council has done remarkable things. You may remember in the old days we used to publish a 'blue book' which told you what fate lay ahead of you for if you committed sins. During Sir Robert Kilpatrick's time as president, the GMC produced *Good medical practice*, and in particular, *Duties of a doctor* which incorporates two phrases which I think are relevant to today's discussions. First, 'it is a duty to keep your professional knowledge and skills up to date', and second, 'that you must recognise the limits of your own professional competence'. Those are probably the only two published Council statements about continuing medical education and professional development.

There are however other activities within Council. In particular the GMC's ability to discipline doctors whose professional performance is substandard has led to the development of tools that have been developed by Professor Lesley Southgate and colleagues. They have been reviewed externally by some world-famous experts in continuing medical education and professional development. What is clear is that we had considerable difficulties in defining what we were looking for until the group went back to *Duties of a doctor* and *Good medical practice*, from which they produced a template which would be widely used to assess doctors whose performance is coming under scrutiny:

- Does the doctor, on average, provide an adequate assessment of the patient's condition, take a good history, reliably elicit the physical signs and then provide or arrange the necessary investigations or treatment and refer, when appropriate, the patient to another practitioner etc?
- Keeping your colleagues informed when sharing care;
- Your prescribing practices;

- Taking part regularly in educational activities that relate to your branch of medicine;
- Taking part in audit;
- Keeping abreast of the law which affects your clinical practice;
- Listening to patients and respecting their views, etc;
- There are issues predominately directed at general practitioners — being accessible to patients when you are on duty, responding to criticisms and complaints (which should apply to all doctors wherever they practise), and then if your relationship with the patient breaks down you make adequate arrangements for somebody else to take over the care.

There are other areas of importance:
- Confidentiality;
- Working in teams;
- Delegation, etc.

These are the items that are going to be used when assessing doctors whose performance is thought to be substandard. My view of life is always that the bottle is at least half full rather than half empty. And we can turn this on its head and say 'Shouldn't we be looking at this as an example either of self-assessment or peer group assessment on a regular basis? Should not these sort of things form the framework of an annual appraisal?' At the moment I am appraised annually by my vice-chancellor in my managerial role within the university. I am also appraised by my head of group in terms of my clinical pharmacology activities. This is an important way forward because it is all too easy and too comfortable to sit in a meeting on a topic I know about already. I should have to participate in activities that are much less comfortable for me in order to bring myself up to date.

PLENARY PRESENTATIONS FROM THE GROUP WORK

Group 1 report
Facilitator and rapporteur, Dr Annabelle Baughan

Question considered by Group 1:

What are your principal recommendations to the following groups to enhance the effectiveness of strategic planning for CME/CPD?

- Trust management
- The royal colleges
- NHS Executive/Department of Health
- Health care commissioners

The group chose to focus on the first three of these.

Recommendations for NHS trusts

The group felt that currently there was no evidence of overall planning for CME/CPD at trust level. The group examined some of the threats faced by NHS trusts in improving their strategic planning. Trusts were urged to realise that planning for CME/CPD is needed because of the pressures of:

- Clinical risk management;
- The increasing need to supervise trainees and how that influenced the time available for consultants; also as a focus in their own development;
- Service pressure in general, but waiting list initiatives in particular.

The group recommended that strategic planning for CME/CPD should not concentrate initially on funding: much more important was to look at the actual activity and content of the CME/CPD taking place. A need for equality of funding with other professions at trust level was seen as both a threat and an opportunity.

Trusts should realise that CPD for doctors should be looked at as a long-term investment not just because the career grade doctors tend to stay in one trust for many years but also because of the need to develop long-term planning for service provision. This tends to be fairly short term at the moment.

A key theme in discussion was the issue of tribalism that Dr Gill had emphasised in his presentation. But the group felt that tribalism was in part a native, instinctive and human response, which would always happen. It was therefore important to look at the uniprofessional wing of CME/CPD and the multiprofessional wing: in other words, to accept that tribes exist and always will and then work to minimise the dangers and the damage arising out of tribalism.

Specific recommendations for NHS trusts to improve strategic planning for CME/CPD included:

- For the trust to realise, admit and broadcast that CME/CPD is a good thing and will improve recruitment and retention of staff and the quality of service delivery;
- To define the objectives of CME/CPD locally and to ask what the trust and its doctors wish CME/CPD to do;
- To take a clear look at the multiprofessional implications of any innovations or change to planning procedures for CPD;

- To define specific local responsibility/accountability for CME/CPD. Whether that takes the form of an individual in a named management role (medical director, clinical tutor etc.) or a director of education or a new group such as a committee, will depend on local arrangements. The responsibilities of that person or group and the accountability of that person or group should be defined. The accountability should preferably be to the trust board;
- To work towards CME planning at directorate level. It was felt that that is the optimum level at which such planning and delivery and care of doctors would happen;
- To make sure that trust systems are supportive rather than punitive;
- To develop a reward strategy for taking part in appropriate CME/CPD. One member of the group felt that extra salary might be included but the rest of the group did not agree. The 'reward' should ideally be exploited at directorate level rather than be part of a pool for the whole hospital. A reward strategy may well be to give time within service for individuals to concentrate on their learning. The group described appraisal as a process that many doctors fear. It was felt very important that appraisal should be positive and part of the reward strategy. For example, if a doctor prepares for and takes part in appraisal, then CME is funded;
- To define the stakeholders for CME/CPD including, for example, health care commissioners, and work with them;
- To look at some way to include non-participating consultants: they are very difficult to find and once found are difficult to support in changing their behaviour;
- To build on the strengths of postgraduate training and to use them to support CME/CPD; for example, an improving culture of training trainees, the infrastructure provided by clinical tutors and educational supervisors;
- For CME/CPD 'champions' to work with the trust to increase the understanding of CPD. Many doctors and many managers do not know what it means;
- To work on clarifying what CME is and what is its relationship to CPD;
- A crucial recommendation is to link the CME/CPD strategy at trust level with recruitment/retention and workforce planning.

Recommendations for the medical royal colleges

The group felt that 'not all colleges are doing the same things. Good things or bad things. So please don't generalise'. The strengths of the current college planning for CME/CPD were perceived as:
- The links with maintenance of clinical and professional standards;
- The colleges have recognised that they need to change — that CME as it stands at the moment is not the ideal system but that the colleges now know that;
- The colleges are still at a very early stage in a new and significant scheme that is still evolving.

Opportunities within college CME planning were identified as:
- Defining what is useful to patients;
- Creating linkage with the individual departmental accreditation that is stemming from inspection of training;
- Looking for ways for the members and fellows to increase their confidence in the colleges which was felt by the group not to be at a very high tide at present;
- Looking at some way of making the colleges' role in CME more supportive rather than inspectorial.

Weaknesses of the current college strategies for CME were identified as:
- They insist on measuring the immeasurable;
- They are not yet signed up to the concept of CPD as opposed to CME;
- The current guidelines for getting CME credits is too prescriptive. Points are not given for certain educationally effective participation;
- The current CME standards are not realistic and need examining;
- Colleges are remote from trusts but as their members and fellows are trust employees the colleges need to link to trusts somehow.

The group identified threats to the colleges' strategic planning for CME:
- Increasing public pressure. Patients are now asking 'Is your department accredited? Are your doctors accredited? Is this hospital accredited?';
- An Australian model in obstetrics and gynaecology, whereby fellowship is withdrawn if not enough CME credits are obtained, was felt not to be the way forward;
- Another threat was the 'OFDOC' body that may be introduced;
- Political pressure for performance management arising from major recent GMC hearings;
- The colleges being forced to compromise on professional standards because college requirements for CME could not be met because of a lack of local funding.

The group's overall recommendation was more a sort of team rallying cry. 'You have made a good start, now come into the real world'.

In summary, the group made the following specific recommendations to the royal colleges:
- CME is only a part. Please develop CPD but bear in mind that CPD is more difficult to measure. Please look into how it can best be measured;
- Be more flexible about what is acceptable for an individual doctor to get credit points.
- However the system develops, do not make it punitive;
- Improve the recording of activity. The group disagreed about whether records of individual doctor's CME hours should be kept at national level. If it is kept at national level, the log books need improving;
- Use college tutors more in a local CME role;
- Look at trainee-related college demands on consultants who are also required to get their CME credits.

Recommendations for the NHSE/Department of Health.

Group members were asked how they saw the current role of NHSE and the Department of Health. Replies varied:
- 'None, it's college business';
- 'Quite a lot is happening. CMO is holding a European conference next March on CME/CPD. The Department will shortly be asking colleges to develop specific CME/CPD curricula. So the Department perceives a specific role in asking the colleges to do that';
- As 'NHS plc', what is your specific investment in CME/CPD as a percentage of, for example, turnover or income? All other successful commercial companies state their human resource investment.

Specific recommendations from the group included:
- Support funding for CME/CPD in some way whether through new money or by making a national statement about hospital clinical contracting;
- Recognise that CME is a legitimate activity for consultants. It is not an escape, it is an appropriate professional activity;

- Recognise that good quality CPD equals good quality people. That is a very important issue about which the group felt strongly;
- Explicitly recognise the tension between staff development and service delivery. A specific sub-issue is that there are some sub-speciality pioneers whose CME is not relevant at trust level. They should have some sort of national funding arrangement.

Ideas for implementation
Ideas that the group members suggested they could implement in their workplace to improve the effectiveness of CME/CPD included:
- 'We are currently within a merger and I intend to look again at the appraisal system we have just designed and make sure that CME/CPD is in there strongly';
- 'I intend to go back to work and set up a strategic group to look at CME/CPD';
- 'I will take a message back to my college. We need to win the hearts and minds of our members and the ownership of CME schemes by the participants is critical. We as a college must be must be more sensitive to local needs as opposed to coming down from on high';
- 'I intend to try and pull together all the tribes internally because we are in it together and we need to look at the multiprofessional aspect of CPD';
- 'I particularly liked the quote this morning "Efficiency is a function of process". And I want to look at local process to allow CME to be universally available to all career grade doctors';
- 'Make happen the work I did earlier this year locally, linking appraisal and CME/CPD'.

Group 2 report
Facilitator and rapporteur, Dr. Peter Wilkinson

Question considered by Group 2:

What are your principal recommendations to the following groups to enhance the support individual doctors in their CME/CPD:

- Trust management
- Health care commissioners
- Royal colleges
- NHS Executive & Department of Health

Two scenarios:
1. No new money
2. New financial investment

Recommendations for NHSE, commissioners and colleges
There was a feeling from government documents that there is still a lack of commitment by **NHSE** to training and education but, in contrast, that planning guidance from the Department was starting to talk about education and training for the first time. The NHSE seems to have finally recognised that these were important areas to comment on but the ideas were rather lost.

One practical idea was that one of the health action zones could test different models of CPD and CME in the community before adopting them in a more widespread way.

There was a feeling that the importance of education has again not been emphasised by the NHSE in dealings with **commissioners.** Commissioners are not recognising at local level that education and training are important. Is it acceptable for them to say that education is important but not provide the money for it? Should they write into contracts a fixed percentage for education? If they did that, there was concern that some institutions or trusts might be constrained from going down particular roads. But cost improvements in an annual trust programme could free up money to improve services through training and education.

The first group anticipated some of our feelings about the **medical royal colleges.** They have been rather rigid in the past particularly about their accreditation of educational topics but they are becoming more flexible. A perception from grass roots level is that the colleges were concerned with income generation here. It was suggested that they could use the money that generated from their members and fellows to push forward local initiatives in CME and CPD development.

The group discussed briefly MOCOMP, the Canadian CME model. This involves the creation of your own educational programme and then entering on a palm top computer what you have done and then feeding that back to the college. There may be initiatives like that which the colleges might test or promote with the funds that they are generating.

We thought that there may be a role within the college regional networks to promote cross-trust education and training — perhaps of use to small trusts. There is a need to get groups of specialists together for external CME and the colleges may have a role in helping individual consultants make best use of that mechanism. This is another example of how the colleges and others should get together. Could there be a meeting of minds with a coherent message coming out to the troops from management, the colleges and the trusts?

Recommendations for NHS trusts

The group made some key points about NHS trusts:

- The importance of the role of the medical director in pushing forward a high profile for CPD/CME within a trust;
- Linking that very much to systems of appraisal;
- Induction is important to set the scene for new consultants joining the trust. The medical director could set up some sort of buddy system — a senior consultant helping a young consultant to get sorted out when they took up their job. Perhaps it would be good to link different specialties — a surgeon with a physician. For example — so they get a different perspective but the main purpose being an introduction to the hospital and the concept of CPD/CME within that hospital;
- Individual doctors are often not seen as working in a team within an institution. Therefore the group had ideas about taking a team away for half a day to look at the needs of the whole team, perhaps sorting out a team CPD agenda. Or perhaps three or four, say orthopaedic surgeons, could sit together and formulate the CPD programme for their unit, sorting out what they are going to spend the money on, how much time they are going to have for this, decide if they need all go to the British Orthopaedic Association meeting at the same time if this causes problems for the service, i.e. develop more of a planning process with a team approach;
- Cross-trust approaches to learning — the colleges have a role but clearly a local approach is important as well;

- The group considered the needs of the 'world expert', the person who does not get involved in local CPD or CME schemes and who may not be affected by what happened within the trust itself.

The group did not talk about money a great deal; it is a 'culture change' not 'cash' which drove many of the group's ideas. We talked about personal development plans and planning for a career change. Hospitals are changing and reconfiguring. People may have to change jobs, to change places or work and doctors should be trained to anticipate this and become flexible in their approach to CPD.

There are fluctuations in demand in our units. Commissioners know that, we know that. When the trust shuts down elective surgery to await the new financial year, why not spend time on education then? There should be surgeons and theatre staff available. It should be possible to find time in the year when you can insert education more easily.

We should tell people what they have taken in the way of time for CME/CPD. If a medical director looks back over the two or three years, it is easy to see that some people have taken many opportunities for CME. But it needs a sense of direction and a sense of planning.

Ideas for implementation

Group members put forward the following:
- 'An appraisal system using medical directors and running through clinical directors';
- 'Looking at multiprofessional groups and looking at their educational needs';
- 'Some kind of appraisal with annual job plans. Looking at CPD and perhaps using a group approach';
- 'Formalising the structure with education and training within the trust';
- 'Professional development plans for consultants starting by April';
- 'Boosting internal training programmes by looking at needs assessment'.

All of these are strong messages about looking at the structure, the way we handle these issues. Appraising ourselves, identifying what we need using the team approach and then planning the whole process. There is not much here about much more money. It is actually using the resources we have to better effect.

Group 3 report
Facilitator and rapporteur, Dr. Jammi Rao

Question considered by Group 3:

What are your principal recommendations to the following groups to enhance the effectiveness of CME/CPD in improving patient outcomes?

- Individual doctors
- Trust management
- Health care commissioners
- Royal colleges
- NHS Executive & Department of Health.

The first point discussed was 'where is the evidence that CME/CPD is linked to improved outcomes?' There is none. However, the group decided early on that if we stopped doing things because of lack of evidence then there was much we would stop doing entirely. Therefore we took it on trust, as a matter of faith, that good CPD, however we define it, leads to a happier doctor and therefore better outcomes.

The next problem was how do you define patient outcomes? We decided to accept that outcomes are linked to CME/CPD and to examine how to enhance this. We arrived at much of the same conclusions as the previous two groups but coming from a different angle.

Recommendations for medical royal colleges

The current practice of CME is motivated not by the individual doctor's desire to do it, nor that trusts demand it, nor that commissioners demand it, but because the royal colleges require it. We made the following recommendations:

The royal colleges should:

- Encourage CME in a non-threatening, non-prescriptive way;
- Encourage local learning initiatives, especially multidisciplinary ones;
- Require evidence of annual self-assessment which should be externally reviewed and verified;
- Define the core skills that each doctor working in hospital requires to perform his/her functions, and the CPD/CME requirements they need to demonstrate as having met;
- Set up a universal system of appraisal and decide about sanctions if appraisal is to be mandatory.

Recommendations for NHS trusts and purchasers

Trust and purchasers were considered together because they were interdependent as far as the finance is concerned:

- Purchasers should ring-fence money — following the model of clinical audit where the funding was ring-fenced until NHSE Working Paper 8 was published. The amount to be ring-fenced was not decided, but purchasers would need to discuss with trusts how it would be dealt with in their spending plans. This would depend on local initiatives and lateral thinking about spending wisely;
- It is important that professionals locally have a say in how the money is spent rather than being the subject of a directive. The focus should be on quality and productivity. Productivity in this context is not just about an efficiency index of throughput, etc., but could also be a function of improved quality;
- Local guidelines are needed on the production of personal development plans and this needs to be linked to the process of appraisal;
- Since trusts and commissioners are the bodies who spend the money they should recognise that there is a definite cost in having a well-trained workforce. People need to recognise that costs are involved and should not duck the issue;
- Doctors in trusts need to be given some kind of incentives to learn as teams rather than as individuals, and to do this on the job. Learning could also be linked to evidence-based medicine and clinical audit rather than a prescriptive approach based on being told what is the best way to do things. Clinical audit has now developed into clinical effectiveness and increasingly this can be linked to CPD;

- The individual doctor should use the appraisal process to negotiate with the trust and peers what new skills and knowledge need to be acquired. Once the system is up and running doctors will be more inclined to come forward to define those areas where they need help, and the trust then has a responsibility to support them. Doctors also need skills in managing their lives to deal with competing demands on their time — social life, art, culture, reading, etc., as well as practising medicine;
- The group suggested getting rid of job plans and replacing them with appraisal and CPD planning. Doctors should accept the inevitability of CPD and take responsibility for defining their own professional development, rather than wait for it to be thrust upon them. It is best to be proactive and to control the process. There is, however, a mutual responsibility for the individual and employer to participate. There is also a responsibility to support colleagues in their CPD needs. The whole process might be perceived as a threatening one, especially for those aged 55 plus, who might wish to take the easy way out to early retirement. We need to guard against a loss of expensive highly trained doctors leaving the service. There needs to be a 'hearts and minds' approach so that people participate as part of the process rather than having things done to them.

Recommendations for the NHS Executive and Department of Health
The group put forward the following suggestions:
- The NHSE should target a small number of areas of action, rather than have broad areas of action such as heart disease. Why not target one particular area e.g. back pain, and link CPD to that? Instead of just publishing guidelines why not include the organisation of training programmes for the management of back pain? At least some action will be taken. It will not solve the whole problem but at least one small area will certainly improve;
- The Department of Health/NHSE could negotiate with the pharmaceutical industry in terms of financing; perhaps in the same way as all finance for R & D is pooled. For drug firms there may be scope for tax relief which could also apply to doctors on their personal contributions. There needs to be an investigation of current funding arrangements and to pool these in some way, to see whether there is money in the system that can go further;
- DoH/NHSE need to recognise the resource implications of CPD. This is not just new money for education but an expansion to the consultant workforce, because there are other pressures mounting up on the existing consultant workforce;
- DoH/NHSE should investigate the clinical audit/CPD link;
- There should be encouragement of multidisciplinary learning especially between GPs and hospital doctors. There are vast areas of clinical medicine that only work if everyone pulls together;
- Workforce planning should not take place in isolation from CME/CPD.

Ideas for implementation
Members of the group offered the following:
- 'Create an education committee in the trust, with an academic adviser';
- 'An awareness of the gaps between the ideal and the reality';
- 'Poor appraisal is worse than no appraisal';
- 'One hospital was reported to have done much work in the field of personal development plans — I will follow this up';
- 'There must be a way of linking personal development plans into the current discretionary award schemes'.

Group 4 report
Facilitator and rapporteur, Mr Frank Quinn

Question considered by Group 4:

What are your principal recommendations to the following groups to enhance the effectiveness of the provision of CME/CPD:

- Trust management
- Health care commissioners
- Royal Colleges
- NHS Executive & Department of Health.

Our task as a group was to look at CME/CPD from the point of view of provision. But it proved very difficult to look at it in terms of the structure of provision without looking at the resources for it, and the uptake, and the factors that conditioned that. So we tended to move around the whole field highlighting some specific and some general issues.

General issues

A general review at the beginning of the discussion revealed the following:

- There was a need to be inclusive, especially to get trusts on board. CPD/CME is not the property of one particular party or stakeholder;
- Trusts, however, do need guidance from the colleges on what they were expecting professionals to do: to know what is an appropriate level of participation and, if it were possible, what is an appropriate level of cost. The process, whatever it is, needs to be both bottom-up and top-down. In other words, it cannot be dictated. It has to be shaped but it should allow room for local endeavour to show and demonstrate itself;
- The 'mandatory' issue needs resolving because there are always people who could still walk away from it and do so. This view was offered constructively as an issue that needs addressing;
- If there are no resources it cannot happen. Resources clouded the whole picture;
- The group identified some responsibilities and the expectations we had of the different parties.

Recommendations for the medical royal colleges

There is a need for a framework and guidance.

- It was pointed out that recently the Royal Society of Medicine had published a complete summary of all the CME proposals and schemes with an interpretation of them. In the interim the Academy of Medical Royal Colleges had done some work in harmonising the core features of CME. But this was not known to many people. And that indicated both a specific need for that particular package to be made widely known and also annually updated;
- It would be useful to get examples of good practice that people would follow because nothing was better than a parable. A parable is good story and you can follow the story;

- An issue was raised about the role of the colleges in conditioning the system to be more receptive to accept training and development. It was noted that where there is teaching of trainees the colleges can intervene to assess the quality of the learning environment. The Clinical Pathology Accreditation scheme can go further than that and look at almost any feature of the service as it is delivered by a laboratory. This must throw up both needs for CME/CPD and the opportunity for it;
- The colleges need to take a wider view on methods, and to devise or commission innovation. But there is a resource and cost implication in this, at least to approve specifications for a wider range of instruments to facilitate local learning;
- The colleges should be active in promoting and encouraging portfolio learning and this would inevitably require personal development planning. It needs local support, but if the colleges do not support it publicly, promote it and offer guidelines, then it is more difficult for trusts or anybody else to take action to support it locally;
- The same applies to mentoring. We had one or two examples of difficulties in mentoring and also some examples of the loss of traditional mentoring. This also highlighted the pressures on consultant time and changes in the working culture. In the past, people would have had somebody to whom to apprentice themselves, who would have supported them over a long period and who would have been able to advise them certainly in the formative years and maybe for longer than that. But the current pressure on consultants and the change in the work structure make that much more difficult to achieve. So if it cannot happen informally, somehow it has to be formalised and included in the structure.

Recommendations for trusts and health care commissioners

The group talked mostly about the trusts because, both directly and indirectly, the trusts represent both their own actions and the consequences of the funding provided by health authorities. So the trusts should see training and CME/CPD in the wider sense as an investment not as a cost. At the moment we tend to think of the problem in terms of sharing the burden of cost and therefore a deduction from other activities. But in the longer term it would be more profitable, more useful, to see it as an investment which enhances the trust's standing.

The group's recommendations to trusts are:
- Provide protected time: this came up again and again. Even if somebody says you can have the time for your CME/CPD, it is hard to take it. The suggestion was made that it should be programmed into part of contractual time, into the 'hard' time. When a doctor is using that time for education, it should be entered in the diary, and it should be inviolate. The doctor should be protected while doing it. Protected time has wider implications too;
- Trusts should facilitate consultants in getting together. The group identified the fact that it was actually harder now for consultants to get together than in the past, and if it cannot happen informally then it should be programmed. In the past the use of 'the Mess' would have been a way of achieving this. Maybe we need to recreate 'the Mess';
- Specify learning time and involve other disciplines. It is no longer adequate or sensible to see this as a closed issue and therefore CPD should be related to the overall structure and strategy of the trust for development;
- CME/CPD is a quality, risk management and recruitment issue. It is not just development. It is not just about going on courses. It is even not just personal review and personal development planning. It is a core feature of the organisational functioning;

- CME funding as a specific issue should be clearly distinguishable from the cost of locums needed to allow people to take study leave. The group did not agree about the mechanism for this because the amounts separated out might get shifted to other budgets. It was agreed that there is an honest and real cost involved in CME/CPD, in whatever form it takes, and that the costs of delivering the service is quite separate. So continuity of service should be recognised in one way and the opportunity and direct cost of CME/CPD should be recognised in another way.

There were two areas that the group felt needed support and guidance from the centre:
- There is a need to identify quite clearly throughout the system money that is to support continuing professional education, and, if necessary, it should be a protected levy on contracts. At a local level it should be clearly identified as a sub-heading, not buried in health authority commissioning contracts with the trust;
- There should be a recognition nationally that more time for education, given the same number of consultants and no other means of expanding clinician time, means (at least in the beginning and maybe for longer than that) increased waiting times or waiting lists and that this is an issue that should be somehow faced quite directly rather than avoided.

Recommendations for the individual
The group was not asked to look at the individual but we found it impossible to avoid this. We identified the fact that individuals have a responsibility for CME/CPD and that it is not just passive participation — something to be done to them. The individual should recognise role changes and new futures and should be encouraged and helped to face up to that. Clinicians are not going to have in the future a 25-year continuous career in the same role with the same kind of job. Perhaps it will be ten years in one role. This will be a challenge and people should be ready for it. But there was a wider range of role options available and there are issues in being prepared to address this. CME/CPD should help clinicians be flexible, not just help them keep up to date technically. They should be active in preparing for change.

Recommendations for the universities
- There are pressures in the university system resulting from the research assessment exercise which uses a points system. In order to get the points and get the money they are having to focus on research and there is a lack of emphasis on teaching. [At the time of the workshop there was concern about the lack of emphasis on teaching. Subsequently teaching has been given a much higher profile following, for example, the publication of *The Learning Age* by the Department for Education and Employment in February 1998];
- There was a suggestion that maybe this is the time for an Open University resource to generate a large mass of the things that people could tap into. It would need to be valid, useful and well designed, and it would also need facilitation at local level.

Ideas for implementation
There are some personal lessons that group members drew from the day. Some of the key ones were:
- The need for protected time for CME/CPD to be built into the job plan so that everybody recognises it;
- A need for local activities to have multidisciplinary features because team working now requires this. CME/CPD can be individualised in some features and phases but not all of it should take place in isolation;

- The idea of the local academic board struck a chord as a means of integrating and putting together all the different expectations — undergraduate, postgraduate, CME/CPD — in the trust;
- Clarifying the meaning of CME and CPD, the distinction between the two and the inclusiveness or otherwise of the concept;
- CPD and appraisal. Many people noted that appraisal seems to be creeping in anyway and certainly consultants are having to get used to doing it for training grades. So perhaps they could they be trained more effectively so that they find it easier to appraise themselves or to appraise other consultants;
- Facing up to the funding issue with the health authority, by saying 'this is the reality, this is what is going to happen, and this is the cost of it';
- Consider using GMC guidelines formatively. The group was struck by the fact that there was a very thorough, very useful and not punitive list. People could use it for themselves as a self-appraisal tool or within a team or between individuals;
- There is a need for mentoring, support and facilitation locally to enable college requirements to be met and married in some way with local requirements. Perhaps the role of the college tutor needs to be looked at again?

Workshop chairman's summary

Professor Cedric Prys-Roberts suggested that the workshop had agreed that CPD and its component CME belongs to the doctor or dentist. It is inherent. It is a moral obligation on the part of the doctor or dentist on behalf of his or her patient. We had also agreed that appraisal is a very important part of the process; and the concept that appraisal could lead to better self-determination of the individual doctor or dentist's requirement for professional development and continuing education. This is a process which involves both self-assessment and peer assessment or peer review.

The message came through very clearly from Professor George that the GMC Guidelines *Good Medical Practice* is a very good model and a template for self-assessment which is probably the best way to approach any form of peer review, whether that peer review is by a senior or a junior, or by somebody at the same level.

We agreed that the colleges have a role at a local level by encouraging the formation of some form of system for self-assessment and peer review, even if their role at national level was no more than just recording activity. A local facilitator for the process of self-assessment and peer review needs to be in place.

We agreed that the process should take place predominantly at a local level rather than at a national collegiate level. Also the trusts and the directorates have the overall responsibility because they are providing healthcare to the patient and that healthcare needs the highest quality of trained and maintained clinician.

The idea of the development of an education or academic board in each trust is an attractive one. It is an extension of what already exists for undergraduate and postgraduate training. Again there are personnel implications in this.

The chairman suggested that perhaps the main message from the workshop was that we need a 'culture change' not 'cash'. The colleges themselves are looking for a 'culture change'. They are well aware of the deficiencies in the present system and that we have to find innovative methods for development. But what are those innovations? We have put forward many today. The colleges will be responsible for standards but they should also perhaps be responsible for generating the concept and the templates for learning portfolios for their specialty, for fellows and members.

And then we come to the NHS trusts, the NHSE and the commissioners. The key message from today is 'What is your investment policy?' I think this is a question we can really ask them. It is no good telling everybody 'Yes, you have got to do CME. We have got to have quality medicine'. You — NHSE, the Department of Health, through the commissioners, through the trusts — have got to provide time and cash to enable the doctors and dentists to do what has already been agreed.

Two final points emerged:
- Should CME/CPD be mandatory? What do we do in the nature of sanctions? Should the sanctions be at college level, at trust level, at a patient level? They are already coming in at a private insurer level. The private insurers are saying 'If you are not on the college's list as having done CME we will not regard you as a proper practitioner'. If the private sector can do it, why can't the NHS do it? It is a question that we will have to address;
- Disappointingly the emphasis throughout today has been almost exclusively on the consultants and not on the non-consultant career grades. They are potentially the weakest link in the system, other than the trainees. Non-consultant career grades must be proficient at whatever level they are going to act and therefore their CME and their CPD needs are just as important as those of consultants.

Continuing education and professional development for hospital doctors and dentists

Giving credit where credit is due:
A study of CME/CPD in three NHS trusts

Soundings Research, June 1998 (Commissioned by SCOPME)

Project team

Bill Fleming, Lesley Golding, Pat Fleetwood-Walker
Soundings Research, Birmingham

Acknowledgements

The project team would like to acknowledge the interest and enthusiasm shown and help given by the doctors, dentists and managers who took part in this study in the three trusts involved. In the midst of demanding professional lives they gave their time generously and deliberated thoughtfully on the issues involved.

Contents

Summary

1. The purpose of this study was to understand the ways in which career grade doctors and dentists in three NHS trusts choose, carry out and evaluate CME/CPD activities. In-depth interviews were conducted with 64 doctors and dentists and one personnel officer from a teaching hospital, from a district general hospital and from a combined community and mental health trust. Dentists from a small department in another DGH were also included. Individuals were interviewed in their clinical and managerial roles.

2. A model of CME/CPD was derived from the interview material. The key concepts in the model were:
    *   The identity of the clinicians involved, i.e. who they are, where they come from, how and where they work;
    *   The ways in which they participate in practice communities throughout their professional lives;
    *   The approaches they adopt to CME/CPD;
    *   Four categories of CME/CPD activity;
        — 'Elective CME;
        — 'Routine activity (mostly work-related meetings);
        — 'Informal interaction with colleagues;
        — 'Learning activity triggered by direct patient care.

3. The interview data was used to illustrate the components of the model. Salient features of the clinician's identity inform their approach to CME/CPD. The major salient features include:
    *   Position in their specialty;
    *   Position in an academic/research community;
    *   Position in the trust;
    *   Degree of sub-specialisation;
    *   Personal circumstances;
    *   Service changes;
    *   Values and principles;
    *   Departmental working arrangements.

4. Approaches to CME/CPD vary, but include:
    *   Pursuing interest in a specialty;
    *   Updating general knowledge and skill;
    *   Pursuing the clinically relevant;
    *   Seeking reassurance;
    *   Giving invited presentations;
    *   Keeping at the leading edge of research;
    *   Filling gaps;
    *   Meeting colleagues;
    *   Maintaining professional pride and esteem;

5. Elective CME activity involves scanning information sources for approach relevant courses, conferences and meetings or scanning meeting and conference programmes to determine if attendance is likely to meet expectations. Many clinicians develop 'a CME habit' which involves a pattern of activity adapted to their particular identity, with minor or major variations depending on changes to salient identity factors.

6. Preferences for lecture style or more interactive formats vary depending on purpose; pre-digested material in lecture format saves time, interactive formats allow for skill development.

7. Many routine meetings are selected principally out of a sense of duty and only secondarily for their potential educational value. Such meetings are more variable in their relevance and effectiveness, but they do tend to cover a wider range of topics than the purely clinical.

8. Informal interaction with colleagues is highly valued by doctors and dentists in this study. Such interaction facilitates the calibration of clinical judgement, reduces the risk of developing idiosyncratic practice due to isolation and facilitates informal 'second opinions' of issues and concerns which arise in practice.

9. Patient care can also trigger educational activity, including seeking second opinions and reading.

10. Regular reading is a major way in which clinicians keep up to date with clinical and/or research developments in their specialties. Reading is predominantly done in doctors' and dentists' own time; involves regular scanning of a relatively small number of journals (three to four) and is usually a mix of general and specialist journals.

11. Enthusiasm for audit has declined over the years. Many doctors and dentists in this study felt that audit is rather unproductive, lacks resources and is not properly organised. Steps are being taken in some places to revitalise audit.

12. Teaching and involvement in postgraduate medical and dental education is recognised as a valuable source of learning for career grade doctors and dentists. Not only does preparation ensure teachers are keeping abreast of developments, but doctors in training also bring with them knowledge, experience and expertise gleaned elsewhere.

13. CME is associated strongly with the colleges' credits and activity schemes. CPD is not a widely recognised concept.

14. Reactions to the CME system vary. Few clinicians consider they have changed their pattern of activity since the schemes were adopted. Many exceed the suggested activity levels by a considerable margin. Keeping log books/diaries up to date is considered irritating by many. A small number of clinical directors sense that levels of CME activity have increased since the schemes were implemented, but do not monitor participation on a regular basis. A few clinicians have found the activity categories useful as guides to what they should be doing. Those who argue that such a system is necessary do so on the grounds that it is there to persuade laggards to keep up to date.

15. CME takes place in a milieu characterised by 'benign community neglect', which provides space for practice communities to flourish and individuals to self-direct their own learning in ways best suited to their needs. CME seems to work reasonably well for most groups of clinicians in this milieu. But benign community neglect can be disrupted for some groups through ignoring their needs, imposing extrinsic requirements, failing to provide adequate resources and denying them access to provider decision making. Most groups in this study experience some of these disruptive influences to a greater or lesser extent, but improvise local solutions. Some groups, e.g. those in teaching hospitals, have access to a greater range of information and financial resources. The most vulnerable groups are those in organisations without a supportive culture and tradition.

Introduction

16. The purpose of this study was to understand how trust career grade doctors and dentists pursue continuing medical education and continuing professional development (CME/CPD), specifically, to find out:
    - How they choose CME/CPD activities;
    - How they perceive access to CME/CPD opportunities;
    - How they judge the effectiveness of what they do.

17. In order to gather their views in depth, the study was carried out in three trusts, a teaching hospital, a district general hospital (DGH) and a combined community and mental health trust. An additional small group of hospital dentists was included from another DGH in order to increase the total number of dentists involved.

18. The trust profiles were as follows:
    A teaching hospital in a large provincial city with 1310 beds, and 400 medical staff, on two sites, two miles apart, one of which backs onto the medical school. Women's and paediatric services are provided by separate trusts in the city. Doctors from these other trusts were not included in this study.

19. A district general hospital in a moderately sized county city with 570 beds and 169 medical staff, on three sites, three miles apart. The hospital provides a full range of acute services for the city and surrounding small towns.

20. A community and mental health trust with 18 medical and dental staff serving a county population of 500,000 with three DGHs. The trust has been recently formed from the merger of two community trusts and mental health services have been transferred from a local DGH.

21. All three trusts are in the same health region, the DGH and community trust being in the same health authority.

22. The additional group of dentists was drawn from a small dental department (four consultants) providing outpatient dental services from a DGH in an adjoining region.

23. A full description of the methodology can be found in Appendix A (page 94).

24. The material from the interviews was used to devise a model of CME/CPD activity. The report describes the model and illustrates its components with material from the interviews. In order to preserve the anonymity of interviewees, where direct quotations are used in the report, we have only occasionally included professional identifiers, i.e. specialty and trust.

25. The report is arranged as follows.

The analytical framework

26. The analytical framework contains a set of key concepts which have emerged during the course of the enquiry. These concepts were derived from the interview material and enhanced by reference to relevant theoretical ideas found in recent literature on practice in professional contexts.

The model

27. Further examination of the interview material was used to derive a model of CME/CPD activity. The model describes the main relationships between the key concepts in the

analytical framework. The model depicts an ideal process derived from the concepts and materials. A number of factors influence the extent to which the model works in practice, as described. These factors are examined in later sections of the report.

Components of the model

28. In this section of the report, the meaning of each component in the model, as understood by doctors and dentists in this study, is illustrated and elaborated by reference to the interview material.

Discussion

29. The final section summarises the main features of CME/CPD to emerge from the study, provides a broad conceptual comment on the model and discusses some of the main factors that can disrupt the ways in which CME/CPD works.

The analytical framework
A. Identity

30. Self-reference ('I') is an ubiquitous, but easily overlooked, explicit and implicit feature of the interview material in this study. This is hardly surprising as the questions asked of the interviewees were about personal activities, perceptions, choices and judgements in relation to CME/CPD, for instance:
    Interviewer: *'Tell me about the CME activities you undertake. What do you do?'*
    Respondent: *'Well, I go to the annual meeting of......'*
    Interviewer: *'How do you decide which meetings to go to?'*
    Respondent: *'I go to the regional association meeting because ....'*

31. During interviews people provide autobiographical information about their personal, professional and organisational lives. As the analysis proceeded the significance of these references to individual identities has grown and come to occupy a central place in the analytical framework and the model of CME/CPD described in the next section. This is based on the evidence in the interview material, which indicates that it is through references to identity that they themselves understand, describe, justify and evaluate their CME/CPD activities. A central concern of the analysis has been to recognise the ways in which features of who the career grade doctors and dentists are helps us to understand their activities, perceptions, choices and judgements. For example, a course, its content and processes are useful and relevant to particular individuals because of who they are and the nature of the work that they do.

32. Notions of interest, relevance and usefulness figure substantially in the material, but only make sense by reference to the identity of the person using them. Implicit in their use is a reference to identity, i.e. interest to <u>me</u>, relevance to <u>me</u> and usefulness to <u>me</u>, and all that this '<u>me</u>' implies.

33. The 'me' to which career-grade doctors and dentists refer has both a static and dynamic significance. It refers to the here and now and the current interaction, influence and significance of personal, professional and organisational factors which delineate 'my current position', together with more dynamic and changing interrelationships between these factors in terms of 'where I have come from and where I am going'.

34. The personal, professional and organisational factors to which the clinicians refer include not only references to circumstances, e.g. family life, professional activities, responsibilities and organisational roles, but also to values, principles, assumptions and beliefs.

35. Thus we have used identity as the emerging organising concept and principle around which the analysis of the material has crystallised, formulating such identities in relation to these interacting and overlapping notions; who they are; where they work; what they do and where they have come from.

B. Participation in practice communities

36. In describing their CME/CPD activities, career grade doctors and dentists refer to a variety of formal and informal, internal and external professional groups, teams, gatherings, associations and societies of which they are a part, with which they interact on a regular or irregular basis, at a variety of local or distant sites and for a range of purposes. These groups overlap with those with whom doctors and dentists work on a daily basis as practising clinicians. Taken together, we have used the term 'practice communities'[8] to refer to these groups. We intend 'practice communities' to include all formal and informal groups to which doctors and dentists belong, or with which they interact during their professional lives, whether convened for clinical, professional, academic, management, social or other purposes. Activities such as individual reading and clinician/patient interaction are also included, as during these events doctors and dentists are still acting as members of professional clinical communities.

37. Such practice communities may have a more or less formal, established, institutionalised or improvised basis, with local, regional, national and international configurations; they may be undergoing slow or rapid change; they may be waxing or waning; they may have a relatively long or short life span and may overlap with other such communities to a greater or lesser extent; they may be broad or narrow spectrum with relatively large or small numbers of active members; and they may reflect more or less strict divisions of labour and be more or less formally convened for particular practice related activities. Medical specialities are a more visible and formal example of such practice communities, particularly significant in understanding CME. Other, less formal, communities often emerge in ongoing practice as participants collaborate for the purpose of achieving practice objectives, e.g. the ward round or case conference.

38. The recent growth in sub and super-specialties in medicine has created a range of smaller, initially rapidly changing, waxing, narrow-spectrum practice communities, some with little local or national critical mass.

39. Identity refers to relationships within these groups and communities. People occupy and change particular positions in social, professional and organisational structures relative to others. These relative positions and their relationships define identities within professional, academic and practice communities.

40. Identities are learned, conferred, maintained, changed, diminished and developed through membership of and participation in such communities. Such communities are also maintained, changed and developed through members' participation in their activities. Each community has a reproductive cycle, involving newcomers joining, becoming increasingly full participants and well-established members then ultimately being replaced by more newcomers.

41. Few of these communities work in isolation; most rely on close collaboration with other communities, both in and out of the workplace.

Reference
8.   Lave J, Wenger E. *Situated learning: legitimate peripheral participation.* Cambridge, Cambridge University Press. 1991.

42.   The knowledge, competence and skill required to carry out the purpose for which the community exists is distributed across community members and between overlapping and interacting communities. For example, the knowledge required to carry out a case conference in psychiatry is distributed among the professionals involved as well as the patients and their family members.

43.   Hence practice communities have developed a range of formal and informal arrangements for managing, maintaining, advancing, displaying, sharing, debating, producing and reproducing the knowledge and skill involved.

44.   Participation in these practice community arrangements, and in their accompanying activities, are the ways in which individuals realise, maintain, change and develop their professional identities and professional competence. Career grade doctors and dentists take part in a wide range of activities, at various sites, as part of their professional practice. Some involve direct clinician/patient encounters but many take place away from the arenas of direct interaction with patients, in libraries, offices, laboratories, dining rooms, meeting rooms, lecture theatres, and conference centres.

45.   A dominant feature of membership of such practice communities is participation in their activities. Being a member of a practice community involves active engagement with its purposes, interests and tasks. In the interview material, doctors and dentists describe a variety of ways in which they participate and take part in the activities of the practice communities which make up CME/CPD activity.

46.   However, they also talk about taking part in, and learning from, a number of the routine, clinical, educational and managerial professional activities in which they are involved, but which they would not ordinarily classify as CME/CPD. Therefore, the analytical framework takes an holistic approach to professional activities, practice communities and participation as the background context against which CME/CPD activity needs to be seen and understood. In this enquiry we have sought to identify the activities through which career grade doctors and dentists consider they learn, and understand this learning against the background of who they are as they participate in the practice communities which compose their professional lives.

47.   There is a strong sense in which participation in the practice communities involves learning. Learning to take part in operations, clinics, case presentations, departmental meetings, teaching, appointment committees, etc, is an integral part of participation in these activities. Participation in the task at hand is the focus of attention. Learning to accomplish the task is an integral part of participation in it. Such 'learning-in-working'[9] or learning-through-participation is a form of apprenticeship,[8] but, for the career grade doctors and dentists, usually without the forms of the master-apprenticeship relationship characteristic of the earlier years of undergraduate and postgraduate medical and dental education.

48.   It is this interaction of identity and participation in practice communities which has emerged from the material in this study that provides the key concepts of the analytical framework, and which has been used to derive the model of CME/CPD. In the next section we outline the model of CME/CPD activity derived from the interview material.

References
8.   Lave J, Wenger E. *Situated learning: legitimate peripheral participation*. Cambridge, Cambridge University Press. 1991.
9.   Seely Brown J, Duguid P. Organisational learning and communities of practice: towards a unified view of working, learning and innovation. *Organisation Science* 1991; 2(1): 40–57.

A model of CME/CPD activity

49. The analytical framework suggests a model with two main components: participation in a range of activities in practice communities, and members of these communities with specific identities.

   Emerging components of the model:
   - Participation in practice communities;
   - Identity.

50. Participation in a specific pattern of activities is both characteristic of, and confers and confirms aspects of a particular identity. For example, taking a ward round confirms the identity of 'consultant' in that specialty and the relationships with other team members.

51. The interview material can be used to add components to the emerging model to show how patterns of participatory activity arise from specific identities. When asked about what motivates and drives some of their CME activities, a number of doctors and dentists indicated an 'approach' to CME, e.g. *'I'm trying to catch up'* or *'I do what I've always done'* or *'I want to be updated'*. In these instances the approach to CME provides a link between identity (who they are) and participation (what they do). To understand what the approach means to them and what carrying it out implies, requires a knowledge of the relevant and salient features of their identity.

   Emerging components of the model:
   - Participation in practice communities
   - Identity — <u>salient features</u>
   - <u>Approach</u>

52. An 'approach' may be used strategically to identify, assess and select specific elective CME activities likely to match the approach. For example, course literature and other information sources may be scanned to identify activities that would enable the practitioner *'to catch up'*.

   Emerging components of the model:
   - Participation in practice communities
         — <u>elective CME</u>
   - Identity — salient features
   - Approach — <u>used to identify, assess and select relevant activities.</u>

53. During this process the approach may or may not be further refined to identify specific learning needs or 'gaps' in knowledge or technique. *'Trying to catch up'* is more likely to generate specific learning needs than *'doing what I have always done'*.

   Emerging components of the model:
   - Participation in practice community activities
         — <u>elective CME</u>
   - Identity — salient features
   - Approach — used to identify, assess and select relevant activities
         — <u>used to identify specific learning needs.</u>

54. An approach to CME/CPD activity can also be motivated by values, principles, assumptions, duties and obligations. Participation in grand rounds, departmental clinical meetings, some local association meetings, teaching and in-house managers' meetings seem to be driven more directly by professional commitment, values and obligations than by strong expectations of their use value in practice. Nevertheless, claims for their relevance

and usefulness are also made, but these are not always the principal grounds on which they are justified. Participation in these activities springs from a more direct relationship between identity and practice community in which taking part is an explicit or implicit condition of community membership. In the model these are referred to as 'routine members' activities'. Reasons for pursuing elective CME can also include issues of principle, but these are often secondary to the use value of the activity selected, e.g. *'I'm trying to catch up'*.

Emerging components of the model:
- Participation in practice community activities
  - — elective CME
  - — routine members' activities
- Identity   — salient features
  - — values, principles, assumptions, duties and obligations
- Approach — used to identify, assess and select relevant activities
  - — used to identify specific learning needs.

55. Another class of activities is those that are triggered by events, issues and concerns arising from direct engagement in patient care, e.g. seeking a second opinion, case conferences prior to ward rounds, out-patient clinics, consulting the literature when a problem arises, raising a case with a colleague over coffee. These can give rise to quite specific, immediate learning needs or an urge to confirm that action taken was the most appropriate in the circumstances. Such patient-triggered activities form another component of the model.

Emerging components of the model:
- Participation in practice community activities
  - — elective CME
  - — routine members' activities
  - — direct patient care
- Identity   — salient features
  - — values, principles, assumptions, duties and obligations
- Approach — used to identify, assess and select relevant activities
  - — used to identify specific learning needs

56. As outlined in the analytical framework, the activities through which doctors and dentists consider they learn are both formally organised, e.g. meetings, courses, conferences and informally improvised, e.g. telephone conversations, corridor conversations, social gatherings. In the model, informal activities have been identified specifically in order to give them greater visibility, in line with the importance attached to them by interviewees. Participation in elective CME, routine members' activities, activities triggered by patient care and informal interaction with colleagues contribute differentially to learning and are valued in different ways by the clinicians in the enquiry.

Emerging components of the model:
- Participation in practice community activities
  - — elective CME
  - — routine members' activities
  - — direct patient care
  - — informal interaction with colleagues
- Identity   — salient features
  - — values, principles, assumptions, duties and obligations
- Approach — used to identify, assess and select relevant activities
  - — used to identify specific learning needs.

57. Clinical and professional work, including CME/CPD, takes place in an environment that impinges on, and provides a context, resources and a policy framework for CME/CPD. The model includes two of the most significant – the royal colleges and the trust – as an organisation.

Emerging components of the model:
- Participation in practice community activities
  - elective CME
  - routine members' activities
  - direct patient care
  - informal interaction with colleagues
- Identity — salient features
  - values, principles, assumptions, duties and obligations
- Approach — used to identify, assess and select relevant activities
  - used to identify specific learning needs
- Environment
  - royal colleges
  - trusts

Figure 1 shows the model in diagrammatic form.

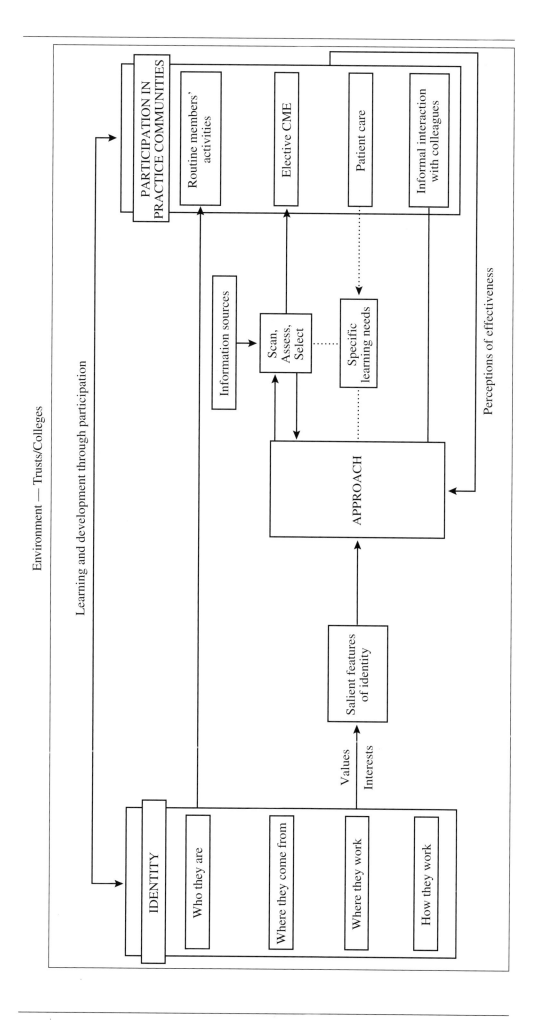

Environment — Trusts/Colleges

Learning and development through participation

Components of the model

Introduction

58. Each component of the model has been derived from the interview material. The purpose of this section is to illustrate what these components mean to the doctors and dentists in this enquiry. They reveal their understanding through the ways in which they make implicit and explicit references to these components. We have used a combination of direct quotations (in *italics*) and redescriptive paraphrasing (ordinary text) to illustrate these components.

Identity
Introduction

59. The decisions individual clinicians make about CME/CPD and the ways in which they judge the effectiveness of what they do depend crucially on their identities. At any one time, particular features of who they are, where they have come from, and where and how they work, become of greater significance and inform their professional judgements of current wants and needs. Who they are, where they have come from, and where and how they work are not mutually exclusive categories. There is some overlap between them. But they provide an heuristic device for describing aspects of identity.

60. The personal, professional and organisational identities of career grade doctors and dentists change and develop through participation in numerous activities in practice communities throughout their careers. Equally, aspects of who they are, where they come from, and where and how they work are key factors in determining their choice of CME activities and in their formulation of reasons for these choices.

Example

61. A consultant radiologist in a DGH had recently returned to the department after a significant absence due to personal, family circumstances. This was at a time when the department had recently acquired MRI equipment and was keen to develop MRI services. The consultant, who was the department MRI specialist, described his approach to CME activities as, 'I'm trying to catch up' and described two specific activities designed to do this. One was a course on a particular MRI technique and the other was a day spent with an acknowledged MRI expert, learning another technique for which no course seemed to exist.

62. In this example the significant identity factors, implicit and explicit in the consultant's account, include:
   - Personal circumstances;
   - Professional perceptions, values and commitments — *'I'm trying to catch up'*;
   - Professional interests and responsibilities — for MRI in the department;
   - Departmental divisions of labour — sub-specialist in radiology;
   - Department objectives and commitments — to develop MRI services;
   - Position in the wider radiology community — able to access a relevant course and persuade a colleague to provide a one-day 'apprenticeship'.

63. *'I'm trying to catch up'* is a professional judgement[10] of need based on an assessment of the identity factors involved and their relative significance at a particular time.

Reference
10.   Fish D, Coles C. *Developing professional judgement in health care: learning through the critical appreciation of practice.* Oxford, Butterworth–Heinemann. 1998.

64. Successful CME activity will change identity factors over time and result in a different judgement of need. Once the consultant considers that he has 'caught up' and the range of MRI services has become well established, this changed identity will inform a different judgement of need, i.e. the relative salience of other identity factors will increase.

65. The professional judgement of learning need and the identification of a 'learning curriculum',[8] i.e. what there is to be learned, is dependent on access to and participation in the arenas of mature practice of various communities, e.g. scanning and reading the journals produced by radiologists and other doctors, reading manufacturers' technical literature, meeting doctors in other departments who request specific radiological services, discussing what radiology colleagues are doing in other hospitals.

66. We have roughly categorised the identity factors to which career grade doctors and dentists implicitly or explicitly allude when talking about CME/CPD as: who they are; where they work; how they work; and where they have come from.

Who they are
Personal circumstances, values and motives
67. A consultant community paediatrician with young children looks for meetings and courses within daily travelling distances to avoid having to stay away from home overnight.

Professional values, principles, motives
68. A consultant rheumatologist tries to identify questions that arise in clinical practice and uses these to guide his reading and literature reviews; a consultant who attends grand rounds acknowledges:
   'But the sole reason for going isn't for me to learn, it is also to be present and to give another view on these kinds of problems for the junior staff.'

Specialism and special interests
69. Many interviewees refer to the relevance of CME activities in terms of the degree to which the activities are specific to their specialism, sub or super-specialty or special interest, both clinical and research:
   'Particularly as a specialist you are expected to know your given field and to have the knowledge at the leading edge of it.'
   'Consultants, once appointed, begin to declare special areas of interest, so we start going to things that relate to that specialism.'

Relative position in the specialty
70. **Newcomers** to the specialty may be up to date but have limited experience, and lack recognition and authority in the specialty. For them, CME is partly about establishing a position and niche in the practice community:
   'One goes to that not purely for the CME but for the social aspects, meeting one's colleagues, feeling comfortable with your own practice by discussion with peers, where they are at and what they think and also learning anything new that is there.'

References
8.   Lave J, Wenger E. *Situated learning: legitimate peripheral participation.* Cambridge, Cambridge University Press. 1991.

71. **Established members** are more likely to be conscious of being potentially out of date but have experience and well-established positions in the specialty:

    'Looking to go to meetings where I want to be updated, where I wanted to know what was happening in that area, where I wanted, in a relatively short period of time to maximise my use of time, to be brought up to date by going to that meeting.'

72. **Leading edge/opinion leaders/innovators** may also be established members, but act as a learning resource for others, but may also provide a focus for challenge by newcomers:

    'I'm a super-specialised consultant in an area that is growing fast. I teach at courses probably more than going to learn myself, but often at conferences I'm talking at, my fellow speakers have things to say that are of interest to me.'

    'There are certain figure heads in certain specialties ..... these individuals are in the limelight almost continuously. Once you have heard them several times ... they have relatively little to say. You don't get the range of diversity of opinion that should be aired.'

73. **Peripheral participants** may be pursuing their own tangential agendas away from the mainstream activities of specialty members.

    'It's the way I am. I'm not terribly social. I think I read and write better than I speak and I think it's probably the way I'm programmed... I'm computer illiterate. I don't have e-mail, etc. People think that's how you should be doing your CME in the future, not sitting with your nose in a journal... The standard lecture is a remarkably inefficient way of getting knowledge in or getting change in practice. It's hard to get excited about it really.'

74. **Old timers** may be recognised and revered as sages.

75. Movement through relative positions in the specialty engenders feelings of belonging, confidence and mastery.

    Relative position in the trust

76. **The clinical director** who recognises that he may be called on to keep the trust up to date with developments in his specialty and therefore needs to ensure he is broadly up to date across the specialty.

77. **The clinical director** who is swamped by management issues and has difficulty finding time for external CME activities.

78. **The clinical tutor** who, on appointment, took a 'teaching the teachers' course which provided a vocabulary for discussing educational issues:

    'Allows you to look at things from more angles' and provides a more constructive way of approaching the role and its requirements.

79. **The staff grade doctor** in A&E who:

    'Carries a bit more responsibility than an SHO. When the consultants are away the staff grade does the review clinic and is consulted by the SHOs.'

    He took a radiology course so that he would be in a better position to confirm a diagnosis when asked by SHOs.

80. **The medical director** who wants to pursue a career in management and finds it difficult to balance clinical and management responsibilities with keeping up to date in his specialty and developing managerial skills and competence.

81. **The consultant,** with general responsibilities in his specialty, but may feel relatively powerless to alter the ways in which decisions are made that impact on his working practice. CME activities have to *'fit in with my life.'*

Membership of professional bodies and associations
82. Such membership may be felt to impose obligations to participate, while also offering opportunities for learning, mutuality, reassurance and maintaining professional cohesion; for example, the Association of Physicians — *'As a member one has to attend at least once every three years.'* On the other hand, such membership may also be partly at odds with the forms of multi-specialty working characteristic of the specialty, leaving consultants feeling they have more in common with members of other professional bodies than their own. For example, an oncologist felt that his college had little to offer his specialty and his links were stronger with members of other colleges.

Membership of an academic community
83. Membership of an academic community affords opportunities and confers obligations to carry out research, the results of which may often be provided as part of formal CME programmes or become available to colleagues through publication. Such membership also orientates members toward leading edge, research based CME activities.

Where they work
Single or multiple sites
84. Working in a single site makes access to a range of learning resources easier, e.g. colleagues, in-house lunchtime meetings, libraries. In contrast, in multiple sites, the need to travel may constrain such access to the point of non-participation, e.g. parking, time. This is particularly the case for clinicians in a community trust whose roles are highly peripatetic. Multi-site working can also increase managerial workloads, e.g. clinical directors, and reduce time available to include a full range of CME activities.

Speed of technological change
85. Working in an environment of rapid technological changes:
    'We are getting new equipment for looking at muscle biopsy measurement. New equipment is an impetus for CME.'

Organisational change
86. Organisational change can create learning and development needs for those involved. For example, where trust clinical directorates are reconfigured in ways which require specialists to adopt generalised roles they had relinquished some years earlier, these changes can generate a perceived need for updating and refresher courses in relation to generalist skills and competence. Equally, trust mergers and service transfers, e.g. mental health services from an acute to a community trust, create temporary culture clashes, increase the visibility of inequalities of opportunity, create uncertainty and developmental 'blight' and disrupt systems. New ways of working and relating have to be learned. New support systems have to be developed. CME may have been given a low priority in view of other changes required. All this may have a temporary 'damping' effect on CME.

Speed of service change and development
87. Rapid service change, for example, during the development of a super specialty, places particular demands on consultants to keep up with the pace of change. This is especially so if they are the local innovators of change, which is also occurring elsewhere.

Proximity to an academic community

88. Being close to, or part of, an academic community provides a wealth of opportunities to consult other experts and leaders in related specialties:

     'I think we are enormously lucky being in a big university institution like this because we have day-to-day opportunities in the corridor or can pick up the phone to another colleague to discuss a difficult or awkward problem with someone else. Just being able to discuss it with someone else makes a huge difference.'

How they work
Working in relative isolation

89. Where career grade doctors and dentists work as single specialists, for example, a lone orthodontist, restorative dentist or diabetes specialist in a DGH, easy access to same specialty colleagues is restricted or difficult. In these circumstances particular forms of CME may be given priority because they compensate for this relative isolation. Without a critical mass, the availability of relevant local meetings may be limited.

Levels of specialism and sub-specialism

90. Career grade doctors and dentists are increasingly identified with progressively differentiated sub and super-specialist areas of interest and divisions of labour, e.g. oncology, surgery, radiology, medicine, anaesthetics. This creates increasingly specialised learning and development needs, but also serves to restrict the range of perceived learning needs to:

     'What is relevant to my area of interest.'

     'I think the generation behind me is very different in that they are becoming much more specialised and eventually people like me who have a generalist background and special interests will disappear. I think, sadly but inevitably, a high-tech area like cardiology and cardiac surgery will become super specialised. We are already seeing that in our own directorate — specialists of little bits of the system.'

91. Super specialists may be few in number, with the practice community very thinly spread throughout the globe. Such specialists need to be able to maintain international contacts. Local and national meetings provide opportunities for teaching but do not enable them to find out what is happening at 'the leading edge.'

92. In a number of service areas sub-specialists are still required to maintain a generalist role or to provide emergency cover, which will often involve working in other areas in the specialty. Maintaining a generalist role as well as working in a sub-specialty can create tensions in relation to CME, for example, an anaesthetist specialising in local anaesthesia for ophthalmic surgery:

     'We're on call for IC but we're not intensivists any longer and the field has changed enormously. It's quite worrying when you go into ICU and you see five or six syringe pumps for a patient — I feel very exposed. But when you explain how out of touch you are the IC specialists say it's all very simple, it's all basic principles.'

93. Sub-specialists can become very anxious when they find emergency working takes them into neighbouring sub-specialities with which they are relatively unfamiliar. Such anxiety can produce clear perceptions of learning need to which consultants may respond in different ways:

     'I was on call at our other site at the weekend and I had a very bad time. The air ambulance brought in two very sick children — both badly injured. I was out of my depth in ITU but I got the consultant on call for this site to come down and give me a second opinion. That's where your learning comes from.'

94. Alternatively, sub-specialists who have always had a general role have developed ways of maintaining involvement in the practice community and pursuing their special interests.

Relationships with other specialties

95. Some specialties see themselves as predominantly providing services to their front line colleagues in other specialties, e.g. pathology, radiology and some aspects of anaesthesia. Such service roles are two edged — requiring sensitivity and responsiveness to the needs and expectations of others, while also maintaining a pro-active educational and developmental role designed to promote the uptake of specialty innovation and change among service recipients. For such internal service specialists CME needs are triggered both by customers' expectations and specialty developments. For example, a staff grade anaesthetist worked with an ENT surgeon who wanted to use a new technique. The anaesthetist had to modify the anaesthetic used as he was no longer able to use a muscle relaxant. He initially used his experience and common sense to make the modifications but checked this procedure with colleagues at a meeting in London and was able to use their suggestions to improve the procedure.

96. Developments in one specialty can lead to changes in the division of labour between specialties:
     'Most of the courses in my specialty of intravascular therapy are concerned with how to put the surgeons out of business.'
     While this may have specific workload and resource implications, it also has an impact on perceptions of CME need.

Where they have come from
Career trajectories

97. Changing roles and responsibilities enhance the perceived significance of some types of CME activity and diminish the value of others. For example, a consultant radiologist due to retire in the near future does not attend any management courses as he has relinquished his management roles.

Benefits of previous experience

98. Some previous experience is seen to be particularly transferable to current work roles and responsibilities, sometimes to the point of obviating the need for further CME in these areas. For example, a clinical director who had learned management skills during a life-long management apprenticeship, in which he had undertaken a variety of management roles, no longer saw any need to attend management courses.

Lack of previous experience

99. Where previous experience is lacking, doctors and dentists can feel ill-prepared for their current roles and seek CME opportunities to fill the gaps:
     'A big part of what we should learn at the beginning of being a consultant is how to train the juniors, particularly as it is all so different from when I was trained. They have to have structured training and teaching and we're not given any guidance in what to do, let alone how to do it.'
     Previous experience, particularly during postgraduate education, can be felt to have over-protected and isolated doctors in training from the 'real' world in which they will have to work.

100. The following brief examples illustrate how identity factors provide an understanding of learning needs and approaches to CME/CPD expressed by career grade doctors and dentists in this study.

Example

101. A consultant in plastic surgery was appointed 18 months ago without previous management and teaching experience. She was surprised by the new responsibilities of her job, particularly the lack of guidance given on management issues and teaching needs. She looked for new ways to develop the service in her specialty. She attended a one-week course in the USA, at which leading international experts in the field were speaking and demonstrating their techniques. Funding was obtained partly from the trust and partly from the company that sponsored the course. Courses to fulfil her needs in management and teaching are not easily available, either because of the paucity of courses or because she is not one of those circulated internally about particular courses, e.g. teaching.

Example

102. A general anaesthetist with three sub-specialisms, who is in mid career. He likes to go to practically orientated small meetings where he can pick up ideas that have a bearing on his practice to *'see how they work for me.'* He avoids big meetings which tend to include material outside his interests. When scanning lists of meetings he asks *'Does it fit in with my life? I don't want to be left behind for professional pride and satisfaction and also because there is a duty to my patients to be aware of changing ideas and changing philosophies.'* He *'scans journals for anything that interests me... occasionally there are some good reviews about topical things which are very good at bringing you up to date.'*

Approaches to CME/CPD
Introduction

103. An approach to CME/CPD can be defined as a general intention, aim, strategy, principle, value or belief in relation to more than a single activity on one occasion, which reflects salient aspects of the identity of the holder. Some approaches are stated explicitly, some we have inferred from doctors' and dentists' descriptions of what they do, or are trying to do, and the reasons they give.

104. An individual may adopt different approaches to different aspects of CME/CPD and these approaches may not necessarily be consistent.

105. As is evident in the interview material, reference to an approach may be used by doctors and dentists in a number of ways:
- To give an account and description of what they do;
- To justify, give reasons for, give an explanation of and account for what they do;
- To provide a strategic direction for choice and action;
- To identify appropriate actions, i.e. in line with the strategic direction, aim or principle;
- To define criteria for choosing and decision making about what to do;
- To define criteria against which the effectiveness of CME/CPD can be evaluated.

106. As indicated in the analytical framework and model, an approach links aspects of the identity of the individual with CME/CPD activity and participation in practice communities. To understand what a specific approach means to an individual, we need to know whose approach it is. For example, *'I'm doing what I've always done'* implies the following:

- Continuation of an established pattern;
- No perceived need to change this pattern;
- That the pattern has been tried and tested and is considered to work, at least, adequately for the individual's purposes.

Such an approach makes sense to an experienced and senior clinician in established positions both in the trust and local, national and international bodies, maintaining involvement with the principal organisations and individuals in a sub-specialty. Nevertheless, this same approach might also 'fit' with other identities.

A number of approaches emerge in the interview material.

Pursuing an interest
107. *'You tend to home in on the sub-specialty you are more interested in.'*
'Subjects that interest me and for which I have a responsibility.'
This notion of interest is more than enthusiasm, i.e. pursuing an interest is about maintaining and developing the part of the specialty in which you work and to which you have devoted considerable time and effort, over many years, to reach the position you are now in.

Pursuing relevance
108. *'Is the subject relevant to my practice?'*

Pursuing usefulness
109. *'Is it going to be of value — will I learn something that I can put into practice or that might be helpful in my research?'*

Following the unfolding story
110. A surgeon likes to attend research-based meetings although there is no immediate relevance to clinical practice, so that when a new technique is developed she is aware of its history and has been able to watch its development and consider its likely impact on her specialty.

Eating fast food
111. *'You try to go to the very carefully pre-digested things, and then you pick anything else.'*

Keeping in the van
112. *'It's about keeping in the van of medical development, keeping in the van of developing, enlarging, bettering medical practice.'*

Being up dated
113. *'Looking to go to meetings where I want to be updated, where I wanted to know what was happening in that area, where I wanted, in a relatively short period of time, to maximise my use of time — be brought up to date by going to that meeting.'*

Not my favourites
114. *'But there are some things I recognise I have to go to, some of the managerial-based things, that I feel, although they are not my favourites, they are not the ones with the hard nutty centres, nevertheless, you have to eat a coffee cream now and again.'*

Seeking stimulation

115. *'Going to meetings wakes your brain up — develops a few new ideas. If you don't go to meetings you sit there in your pond and you don't get stretched and stimulated enough. I find you are always a bit brighter, you've got a few new ideas and attack your work with a bit more zest.'*

Reconnoitring

116. *'I read, I talk to people, I go to meetings and therefore get a feel for what's important and what isn't, what's developing and what isn't and put that against the background of my own activities and roles and then, try, where necessary, to fill the gaps.'*

Seeking reassurance

117. *'Want to know what other people are doing in other centres — am I doing it right? Are there ways I can improve what I am doing?'*

Improving teaching

118. *'I have been looking out for every opportunity to see how I can teach better.'*

Visiting the trade fair — (British Geriatrics Society)

119. *'I like to go — it's the trade fair.'*

Making up the points

120. *'Frankly, I do it to make sure my numbers are up, that I can tally up the requisite number of hours, because this is the sort of stupidity that the system demands if I'm not to get a self-righteous letter from Glasgow.'*

Learning from colleagues

121. *'Discussing your particular area of work, your particular specialty, is very useful and stimulating and does change what you do.'*

Going to the source

122. *'I look for courses where a new technique has been flagged up in the journals and the originator is speaking.'*

Challenging the gurus

123. *'The problem with all these meetings is that the people who shout loudest get heard and sometimes what they are shouting about is not necessarily the right view and it is important that other views are stated. So it is important that one participates, so I try to put my point of view.'*

Being in the A team

124. *'You don't want to be thought of as a member of the B team.'*

Shopping

125. *'I have a mental shopping list — it's not large.'*

Patient driven reflection

126. *'I could argue that the ward round I have just done was CME. There are some interesting cases and I've learnt things from them. It stretches the mind as to how to deal with them.'*

Avoiding the irrelevant, unhelpful or boring

127. *'I choose to ignore things that are boring.'*

Having nothing better to do

128. *'I occasionally go to the Tuesday radiology meeting, frankly when I haven't anything better to do, because I don't think I learn very much.'*

Filling gaps

129. *'If you feel it is something lacking in your previous background that you need to know about then you'll go, to feel whole as it were.'*

Invited

130. *'I've been lucky enough to be asked to a very special meeting.'*

Attracted by gurus

131. *'It could be a meeting where you know there are certain experts going ... you think, gosh, that's worthwhile going to.'*

Meeting obligations

132. *'Society meetings — they are not compulsory, but you feel you ought to go to them because they are the professional society of your specialty... there is strong professional pressure.'*

Increasing knowledge

133. *'Subjects that I do know and I'm interested to see what other people think and the subjects that I do not know and would like to know what is going on.'*

Problem solving

134. *'They might hold the answers to some of the problems encountered clinically — small areas of concern where you wonder how someone else gets round that.'*

Pursuing what catches the eye

135. *'Just happened to see something ... and thought, I must go to that.'*

Developing services

136. *'Something came up fortunately at the time when we were seriously beginning to develop the service.'*

Watching the pennies

137. *'If a drug company puts on a relevant meeting that is interesting and free you are more likely to go to that.'*

To meet old friends

138. *'You meet your old friends, you've taken examinations together and at lunchtime you grumble about how things are going wrong with the management and see that everybody has got the same problems.'*

Going places

139. *'My approach to conferences now is that I'm going to go to the ones that are nice places — social-wise. I go to the London ones because my daughter's a nurse in London. I went to Chester because I've never been there and I went to Windermere because I've never been to the Lake District properly, that's how I look at it.'*

To support career moves

140. *'I reached the stage where I needed to gain some management experience for my CV.'*

141. While we have not included here a full analysis of the roots of each of these approaches in the identities of the individual doctors and dentists concerned, these additional examples further illustrate the value of understanding these approaches, not as disembodied objectives or perspectives, but as principled intentions arising from salient features of who they are, where they have come from, and where and how they work.

Example

142. An orthopaedic surgeon with super-specialty, in mid-to-late career, who is a college tutor and teaches. He has a regular pattern of CME activities related to his super-specialty, which he follows from year to year. He is attracted to courses where good speakers address his special interest, where the subject is one he either has not heard of before or has been flagged up by the journals as something new and the originator of the technique will be speaking. He wants ideas that he can put into practice. He does not attend college meetings as he feels they do not cover his specialised field sufficiently. As a result he has to travel further afield for his CME, e.g. Europe. Occasionally he attends generalist meetings for the interest and to keep up to date. He values contact with colleagues and is highly selective in his reading, including research and review papers.

Example

143. An experienced psychiatrist who works in the community. His approach to CME is informed by a philosophy of psychiatry as *'a soft science'* where *'innovation is often down to one person. Development in psychiatry is not driven by a linear, logical process. Someone may have a wild idea that turns out to be right.'* His CME activity involves looking for ideas, both to develop his clinical practice and his ways of working. *'You get a lot of new ideas from colleagues who have read something you haven't, or done something you haven't or trained in something you haven't.'*

144. These approaches also suggest ways in which individuals intend to participate, in and engage with, the specific practice communities to which they refer. For example:
   - Going to same specialty meetings to find out what other people think or what other people are doing.
   - Going to specialty conferences to *'pick up the carefully pre-digested things'*.
   - Going to practical courses to learn new techniques from experienced clinicians.
   - Attending meetings which give a different perspective on a technique because *'they might hold the answers to some problems encountered clinically — small areas of concern where you wonder how someone else gets round that'*.
   - Learning from reviewing papers for journals.

145. Some are more readily identifiable as approaches to learning or expressions of learning style/preference than others. Some preferred to be lectured — *'Sit me down in a classroom and tell me things'* because it was felt to be an effective use of time. Some felt they *'learned more at the meal than at the meeting'*. Others wanted interactive or hands-on experience of techniques.

CME/CPD Activity

Introduction

146. Participation in practice communities refers to all the formal, informal, internal and external clinical and non-clinical activities of doctors' and dentists' activity in their capacity as members of their profession. CME/CPD is a subset of these activities.

147. When describing their CME/CPD activities, doctors and dentists in this study referred to what they do in a number of ways, summarised succinctly by one consultant as:
'I read, I talk to people, I go to meetings.'

148. In the model, we have used a rather different classification of these activities to highlight relationships with identity, approach and participation as referred to by the clinicians in their interviews.

149. **Routine members' activities,** e.g. grand rounds, teaching, departmental meetings, etc, are part of the daily, weekly or monthly round, some more deliberately convened for educational purposes than others and affording opportunities, in varying degrees, for deliberate and incidental learning.

150. **Elective CME** includes those activities deliberately selected for education and training purposes.

151. **Patient care** refers to formal and informal learning opportunities afforded by direct clinician/patient interaction. Such learning may be apparently incidental:
'You're learning all the time. Five minutes with an interesting patient edified me this morning,'
or sought deliberately:
'Interrogating MEDLINE on the basis of questions that have been raised in my clinic.'

152. **Informal interaction with colleagues** has been included because of the value interviewees placed on learning from each other. Such dialogue takes many forms and occurs on numerous occasions, both in clinical work settings and in spaces created during routine members' activities and elective CME. We have included reading as part of such informal activities because it involves indirect, rather than direct, communication with, and in, practice communities.

153. When describing CME/CPD activities, doctors and dentists often included an evaluation of how effective, useful, relevant or valuable they considered the events to have been. The following account of their activities therefore includes these evaluations.

Informal interactions with colleagues

154. Routine clinical work may or may not provide opportunities for impromptu, informal interactions with colleagues, from which clinicians can learn. Where clinicians routinely work closely together in ways that allow frequent, unplanned interaction, e.g. radiology, they have many opportunities to consult each other in a system of ongoing, on demand, needs led, informal, peer review by checking each other's radiographs. Some clinicians commented on limited opportunities for such interaction, for example, in anaesthesia where a lone sub-specialist anaesthetist will be working in theatre, without doctors in training and without colleagues with similar sub-specialty experience to call on. Increasingly, work schedules also limit the time available for informal discussion and entail consultants working on their own rather than with colleagues:

'Contact with colleagues is extremely valuable. It is a tragedy that the working day has become so filled, that working with one's colleagues has been more or less destroyed.'

155. Such contact with colleagues is highly valued:
     'Through professional conversations with colleagues, in reality that is how, mostly, how you learn as a doctor.'
     'Discussing your particular specialty, which is useful and stimulating, and does change what you do.'

156. Informal interaction with colleagues created during meetings, courses and conferences are equally valuable:
     'I learned more at the meal than at the meeting.'

157. It is on such occasions that temporary, improvised practice communities emerge which enable peers to recount stories, compose approaches to practice, gain reassurance and overcome the dangers of developing idiosyncratic practice due to isolation:
     'I think if you are not interacting with other professionals in the same field your clinical judgement can go wildly awry. You need some sort of calibration of your clinical judgement and that needs to be fairly continual.'

158. Some clinicians in the study saw the maintenance and development of clinical judgement as a matter of experience, initially learned through apprenticeship and continued through learning from mistakes and successes. All emphasised the value of contact with colleagues and the dangers of professional isolation. For some there is an element which may be innate or a result of your initial training — the ability to assess patients. The second element is judging the appropriateness of particular clinical practices for particular patients — and that is refined through CME.

159. The mentor system in psychiatry was cited as a good example of a more systematic approach to fostering interaction between colleagues and providing mutual support.

Routine members' activities

160. Doctors and dentists attend a variety of regular or intermittent local, regional and sometimes national meetings that they often feel they should support out of a sense of obligation or duty to colleagues and clinicians in training. Some of these are contractual obligations. These meetings include journal clubs, grand rounds, case presentations, audit meetings, specialist associations, regional research groups, covering clinical, sub-specialty, management, medico-legal and professional-political topics. The format is predominantly lecture presentation plus discussion. Some also include a social component, perhaps with a pharmaceutical company contribution towards a meal.

161. The career grade doctors and dentists commented on a number of issues related to these routine activities:
     - Relevance, either to *'my practice'* or *'my interest'*, is often unpredictable and a matter of what happens to be on the programme for the day.
     - Quality varies with regard to the presentation skills of the speakers and their ability to maintain the attention of the audience.
     - More rarely, clinicians commented on the quality of the content, for example, reports of poor-quality research or audit projects.
     - Benefits vary, in terms of learning, some rated highly, others considered to be largely repetitious.

- The range of topics varies, both within and beyond subjects of interest or relevance to the interviewee concerned. For some diversity is a positive feature:
  'I learn most from topics with which I am not familiar.'
- Attendance and access:
  'I don't go as often as I should.'
  'If it's a 6 o'clock meeting in Q (50 miles away) and my clinic finishes at 5 o'clock, I'm unlikely to get there.'
- Cost:
  'There is no funding for these, so we have to find ways to keep the cost down.'
- Reservations about pharmaceutical company sponsorship.
- Value in maintaining contact with colleagues, rated particularly highly by lone consultants, e.g. a single DGH orthodontist; rated less highly by some academic clinicians and super specialists whose elective CME is substantially at a national and international level.

Elective CME/CPD

162. Elective CME is predominantly a provider driven system in which choosing is marked by a range of scanning, browsing and monitoring strategies designed to select from the mass of what is available that which will match a set of more, or less, clearly defined criteria. Such scanning may be designed to include some possibilities and exclude others. These criteria are often rather broad, informed by an 'interest' in a specialty or particular area of 'special interest'. More rarely is such scanning directed by a single, specific, clearly identified need.

163. Such a selection process happens at a number of levels; identifying an approach relevant event, e.g. gap filler; assessing the potential of the identified event to fulfil the approach:
'I look for a course covering areas of my work where I think I can benefit from updating myself. If I was conscious of the fact that children with kidney problems was an area that my knowledge was a bit shaky on, and I saw a course advertised on it, I'd write off for the details and if they looked interesting enough, then I would apply for it. If the course looked like a series of dull lectures by a series of dull people, I wouldn't go. How the course is sold by the people organising it is fairly important.'

164. Preferences for length of course and location also figure in the decision:
'In choosing external courses I look to include how long the course is. I prefer two-day courses because they are packed with information, and in London, including an overnight stay because this allows me to talk to colleagues. I don't go purely for the didactic elements of the CME, but for courses or conferences that are applicable to my practice. I don't choose pure research. Who is speaking tells you a lot about the content and whether it is research or clinically relevant.'

165. Meeting programme guides are one source of information about quality and relevance:
'What I look for in deciding which conference to go to is what the programme guide says. Most conferences have a reputation and you know what is likely to be going on before you get there.'
'You look at the programme, for example, I'm a member of the British Pharmacological Society and I almost never go because I go through the programme and I say to myself, which of these particular talks is going to be of benefit to me? And usually I don't go because I come to the conclusion that it's not terribly helpful.'

166. But meeting programme guides can be inadequate or misleading:
'I went to a meeting where the agenda looked good but when I got there it was much more orientated towards workers outside health.'

167. For some clinicians, part of their annual CME activity becomes a standard pattern:
'I have a pattern of CME in my mind and it's a regular pattern from year to year. I think people tend to get a regular pattern at age 40 which they then keep.'

168. The pattern can change over time as salient identity features change:
'In fact I'm bored with the British Society of Rheumatology, I've been going for the last 12 years and I'm not going to go this year. I've started to go to the American College of Rheumatology five-day meeting. The amount of information and the quality is at a much higher level because it's very much an international meeting rather than a national meeting.'

169. Some meetings are almost automatically included because they are the 'annual jamboree' of an association or society — the 'trade fair' or are the only national, European or world gathering devoted to a sub- or super-specialty at which the known experts will be present.

170. A few clinicians in this study feel the process of choosing relevant and useful elective CME activities is rather *'ad hoc'*, being unpredictable, unsystematic and very much dependent on the whims and fancies of providers; *'It's like swimming in custard'*. Others seem to be able to chart a more purposeful and focused course through the jungle, avoiding the swamps of time wasting, irrelevant, boring and poor-quality activity.
'I knew what the subject was. I knew what the lectures were going to be and I knew that the speakers would be good and it was all about stuff that was relevant to my branch of medicine.'

171. Factors that made for this difference seem to be:
    - The clarity and specificity of wants and needs;
    - The availability of accurate, detailed and timely information from providers;
    - Sufficient familiarity with the practice community and its membership to be able to assess the relative position and significance of contributions and therefore their likely value;
    - Knowledge of the presentation skills of speakers.

172. The majority of elective CME/CPD activities chosen by doctors and dentists in this study were specialty related. Interest in and selection of other topics, e.g. management or education, was limited. A small number of clinicians had attended equal opportunities courses organised by the trust and found them very revealing, highlighting actions and behaviours the consultants had not noticed in themselves nor recognised as displaying bias.

173. Responses to management courses were varied, but on the whole rather negative:
'I tend to avoid those.'
    - Recently appointed consultants who were grappling with management issues recognised their needs, but could not find an appropriate course or felt that management skills and competence could not be learned from a course. Some felt their previous experience in managing research teams and projects had given them the necessary skills.
    - Experienced clinicians who had taken on a variety of management roles over the years felt they had thereby developed the necessary skills and competence.
    - There were those who felt management courses were still grounded in commercial philosophy alien to the ethos of health care.
    - Those who attended management seminars, largely as part of a management role, e.g. clinical director, found them valuable because they addressed issues outside and beyond familiar territory.

174. Responses to courses on education and teaching varied, but were, on the whole, more positive:

- Some had taken such courses as a requirement of their appointment and found them very useful, particularly the opportunities for active participation with video and other feedback;
- Two were taking M.Ed. courses arising from a special interest in medical education and a desire to improve their teaching;
- Some, e.g. clinical tutors, were included in a regional strategy to 'train the trainers' and found the short courses of value in developing their thinking about educational issues;
- At least one newly appointed consultant wanted to attend the 'training the trainers' courses but could not as priority was given to clinical tutors and course organisers;
- Some found the 'group work' format of some education workshops less than helpful:
  'But if you look back at the end of the day — I spent six to seven hours there and what did I actually learn for my effort?'
- Newly appointed consultants who were given opportunities to teach during their years as doctors in training were less likely to feel the need to attend courses on education.

175. The doctors and dentists varied in the extent to which their elective CME activities followed an established pattern. Sub- and super-specialists and academic clinicians were more likely to have developed a pattern consistent with maintaining involvement in and with the key community groupings in their areas of interest. For many in this category, elective CME means being an invited contributor to these events. These consultants and academic clinicians are often members of insider groups around which the community is built.

176. Other clinicians, less centrally involved in such practice communities, may attend a smaller number of regular external conferences, such as the annual college or association meeting, and select others on the basis of specific clinical relevance or *'what catches my eye.'*

Patient care

177. Improving patient care is the principle that underlies the approaches and activities described in this study. More specifically, caring for patients is perceived as a learning experience and triggers different types of educational activity.

178. **Caring for patients as a learning experience**
   'Individual patients can be a great learning experience.'
   'Education doesn't have to be formal — a lot of patients can be educational. I could argue that the ward round I have just done was CME. There are some interesting cases and I've learnt things from them. It stretches the mind as to how to deal with them.'

179. **Patient care as educational trigger**
   'Most of what I acquire is done through MEDLINE searches, interrogating these facilities on the basis of questions that have arisen in the clinic. I can give you plenty of examples of questions that have arisen recently in my practice and haven't had sufficient information in the textbooks, so then I have needed to do a formal search.'
   Such facilities are not yet available in the community trust, although there are plans to develop them.

180. Patient care also triggers requests for second opinions, informal telephone and face-to-face discussion with colleagues and other specialists. In this study the opportunities to do this were perceived to be greater in the teaching hospital than in the DGH and significantly reduced for some lone super-specialists and some highly peripatetic clinicians in the community trust.

Reading

181. Doctors and dentists in this study identified reading as a key element in keeping up to date:
'I do think the most important thing is probably keeping abreast of current literature. The best way to keep up to date is by reading current literature and articles and looking at what other people are doing and saying, "That looks like a good idea, I'll try that on my next case".'
'I learn a lot more from reading than from lectures.'
'Reading journals is probably the next most profitable thing [after going to meetings]. On a regular basis I keep up to date in that way.'

182. They scan a combination of journals and specialist journals:
'I take the British Journal of Anaesthesia, the Association of Anaesthetics Journal, the BMJ, the British Journal of Hospital Medicine and the Royal Society of Medicine Journal. If you read those, you've got your specialty and your general journals.'
'I scan the BMJ, the Lancet and JAMA each week. I read in full only the papers that are related to my special interest or seem relevant to something in my clinical work.'
'I read the college journal and the BMJ and pick up what is interesting and topical — it's directed by what is interesting and useful. I do a literature search to find out more about the areas in which I'm interested.'

183. What is read and how much depends on interest and relevance to their clinical work:
'I'll read the leaders that relate in a broad sense to what I do. I'll read original research and review articles that are actually relevant to the patients I treat or fundamental understanding of what I do. I scan through correspondence — a lot isn't relevant.'
'I take and read three journals a week. I don't read them from cover to cover. I go through them and read all the things that are relevant to me. For some things I read the whole article but some things I just read the summary. For lots of things there is a three-to-four line take-home message.'

184. Reading will not always be limited to one's own specialty:
'You're more likely to read what grabs you straightaway, but that doesn't necessarily mean that you just read what's in your specialty. There are more thoughtful articles in the Lancet from individuals that take a completely different slant on an area and which are also very instructive. So you read the title and you try to read between, you flick through and sometimes you pick things up and actually just by scanning the front page with the articles in it you pick out things that you wouldn't necessarily think that you would.'

185. Things of relevance to colleagues may be read and passed on:
'I scan through the BMJ and the Lancet on the day they arrive. If I think there is anything really world shattering that might be of great importance to me or of special interest to people in the department, then I'll get that photocopied and sent to them and I usually keep a copy if there's something that I'm interested in.'

186. For some clinicians, review journals are particularly useful:
'There are some very useful journals which provide a summary of the topic — it is easier to read if the author is summarising his/her area — saying what should be done.'

187. Others combine research and review:

'I am selective, choosing research papers and some review articles giving the latest on a particular topic — from refereed journals, not the popular journals.'

188. Some have quite particular reading patterns:

'With the BMJ I look at the list of the contents, then the editorials, then I start at the back. I start with Minerva, look at the soundings, look at the names of people in the obituaries and then go back to the front. I look at the detail of an article and try to work out where it fits with the bigger framework. Often it gets put to the side to get dug out six months later. If I'm happy that I have read everything I find interesting it is filed in a box and will probably never be looked at again. Sometimes I make notes on an article I think is interesting. I make out a card with the title and the main points of the article. If I'm not happy I have read everything, if there are one or two things I think may be interesting, but I don't have time for at the moment, then it gets put on a pile with other BMJs and journals and every six months I take 10–15 off the pile and have a look at them. But I never get to the stage where it completely disappears, there is always a sort of backlog.'

189. Finding time to read is a major difficulty:

'I don't actually have enough time to read in the depth that I used to. I used to read all the journals that are relevant to make sure that I had read every journal so that I was fully up to date with what was published.'

190. Predominantly, reading is done 'out of hours':

'I read the journals but I do not consciously set aside time to do so — I usually read them over a cup of coffee after dinner — in my own time.'

'I come in on the bus and that gives me a chance to sit for 25 minutes and read and if I go home on the bus I can manage to read three journals that way in a week. Nevertheless I still fail to keep up because they get stacked up and you sometimes end up with a pile of 15–20 to get through and then you're quite ruthless about what you read — you cut corners all over the place and read lines and get a message and throw the journal away.'

'I drive my wife potty reading the Lancet and the BMJ.'

'I probably skim stuff on a Saturday morning when the children are watching TV — I've got half an hour so I'll have a quick read of that or one evening you might pick up the thing. I don't have time during the day to read journals so they all end up here under the desk.'

191. Access to libraries is variable, as is the availability of MEDLINE and other electronic resources. Community clinicians who work near, or also have joint appointments in, the local DGH, have access to its library or postgraduate centre. Others have much more restricted access. In the teaching hospital, pressure on the medical school library by undergraduates and researchers is necessitating development of better facilities in the hospital.

Audit

192. We asked specifically about clinicians' participation in audit and its value. Views differed. The importance of audit in principle was mentioned by some:

'I think this is an aspect of CME. Equally, I see it as part and parcel of clinical practice as well. How we got away in the past with doing things, and never bothering to look at how well we were doing, amazes me.'

193. But in practice, enthusiasm for audit seemed to be waning…..
This is not an atypical view of audit as perceived by many of those interviewed:
'General surgical audit meetings, which are compulsory according to the college, seem to be a total waste of time and badly attended — that's people voting with their feet. They find that at 8 o'clock in the morning they are not going to get out of their beds for something that is a total waste of time. Occasionally there will be a speaker who is presenting something that is of interest or someone who has done a decent audit project and you actually learn something from it — but they are few and far between. Tends to be a fair bit of number crunching of the old type of morbidity/mortality meetings — people very much on the defensive, trying to justify their actions. Poorly attended by juniors who should learn something from it and by consultants who should be asking the questions and trying to stimulate the discussion. There is no organisation at all as far I can gather. Before audit was the "in" word we had morbidity/mortality meetings. Audit became that meeting. For many firms it has gone on in exactly the same mode, but it's not audit.'

194. …..sometimes to vanishing point:
'I think I'm meant to get involved in audit but I haven't noticed much of it so far.'

195. In some areas, measures are being taken to revitalise audit:
'Audit got a bad name in the past because when it indicated a need for a change in practice it petered out at that point. Often it was difficult to get one's colleagues to change…. What is needed is a more systematic review of the way things are done — it's a far more open and multi-disciplinary process.'

196. Constraints of time, resources, support, resistance and quality assurance conspire against effective audit:
'Because of pressure of work, apathy, self-righteousness and fatigue it is quite hard to get people enthused to look at the standard of what they are doing.'
'Difficulty is trying to make audit exciting. There is a problem with having audit meetings too frequently because you can't maintain the excitement, but if you don't have them frequently enough, people forget about them.'
'Audit is a required exercise — difficult to run with the time and resources available. You really need an autonomous audit co-ordinator — without that you probably end up worse off because you play at it.'
'Should be better but it takes a lot of time to prepare things for the meeting and that's probably what the limiting factor is.'

Learning through teaching

197. A number of specialties in this study have training posts. The career grade clinicians involved acknowledge that teaching and contact with doctors and dentists in training provides learning opportunities in a number of ways.

198. Teachers must be up to date:
'Most clinicians take their teaching very seriously and it's a learning experience — to teach you must learn.'
'One of the most useful learning experiences for me is, on a regular basis, having to teach other people.'

199. Teachers can learn from their 'juniors' and ' students':
'It's nice to have a trainee to learn from and to teach at the same time.'
'I learn more about arrhythmias from the journals, or more importantly the juniors.'

'Last night I marked five essays for third-year medical students on CJD. They were super reviews — absolutely up to the minute. I learned more about CJD from those than in reading.'

200. Teachers can be challenged by 'juniors':
'My interaction with students and juniors — the contact with fresh minds that are relatively green to ask questions that to them seem obvious, but which I can't answer. So teaching is as important to me as it is to them.'

Preferred ways of learning

201. Enthusiasm varied for the lecture method which still dominates many formal CME activities. In support, some clinicians stressed the time-efficiency of lectures and the advantage of having someone else organise the material.
'Sit me down in a classroom and tell me things. Time is limited. I know educationalists are encouraging self-learning, but in practice I'm not all that good at being self-disciplined. So I'm better knowing that for three days I'm going to be sitting in a formal course where they will teach me solidly for three days. That's the most effective use of my time.'

202. Others echo such an apparently passive approach:
'I would be looking to go meetings where I want to be updated, to be brought up to date.'

203. Others stress the value of having information *'sifted'* and presented in *'digestible form'*. 'That is what good meetings do', i.e. save busy clinicians time reading and reviewing journals.

204. Informal, interactive methods are preferred by some:
'Although I lapped it up as a student, I don't personally like a lecturing approach. I prefer something that's more informal where there is more scope for discussion that's not a formal talk. And the days I think I enjoy most are days that combine some formal lecturing with some workshop types to it, with more participatory learning. I think they get more out of it by participating.'

205. Other interactive methods also appealed:
'The ATLS type of courses are great fun. They have a large practical element to them.'
'Interactive sessions are good, for example, a "how to teach" course where there is audience participation. You have a discussion and someone has to present the findings of the group. That's quite a good way of learning.'
'Another interesting way is hands-on, where you have to do things with a manikin and you're assessed at the end of three days. That's a really super way of learning.'
'I participate in a sort of case meeting on the Internet, where cases are presented and you respond with what you think the possibilities might be and how you would proceed with the investigation. It's the most valuable thing I've found.'
'Informal discussion with colleagues is one of the most valuable forms of CME. We get together once a week in our department to discuss all aspects of our work — audit, management, staffing, departmental commitments and clinical matters — extremely useful, opinion forming.'

206. The patterns of CME/CPD vary in the emphasis and value placed on different types of activity. Some give greater weight to reading, others to local meetings and still others to international meetings. As with the selection of individual activities, this pattern reflects who they are, where they work, how they work and where they have come from.

Constraints

207. The model identifies key features of an ideal process, i.e. it draws a road map rather than describing road conditions. While for some career grade doctors and dentists the model/map is an adequate representation of CME/CPD processes, for others more detailed consideration needs to be given to the contingencies with which road users have to deal. There are a number of ways in which CME/CPD in practice can fall short of the ideal depicted in the model. For some individuals, the journey hardly begins before they run into difficulties. For others, the end is in sight before serious misgivings arise. Some are able to improvise solutions, compensations and work arounds; others have to abandon the trip or try again another day.

208. A number of constraints may make access to some CME/CPD activities difficult or impossible, or reduce motivation to participate.

209. CME/CPD takes time, which is in short supply:
'There are some offers of management courses but I can't take them up — I haven't got time to keep up with my own stuff.'

210. Service commitments may have to take priority:
'If it's my week for 'take' then I can't go.'

211. Courses on particular topics may be oversubscribed:
'They are very difficult to get into — by the time I apply, the places have gone, but I do then get first refusal when the course is repeated.'

212. Course providers may not give sufficient notice.

213. Family commitments may make attendance difficult or impossible:
'With a family, going on residential courses is difficult for me. I try to look for courses that are a day course or where I can commute on a daily basis, that mostly means courses in the region.'

214. Meetings may be too far away to be worth going to:
'If you're going to go some distance then you really want more than one lecture that is going to be good. You really want a series of lectures and you want good, recognised speakers who you know will speak well and can actually bring you right up to date.'

215. Travelling between sites may take up half the meeting time:
'I am never in the hospital at lunchtime because my morning and afternoon clinics are in different places so I have to use lunchtime for travelling so this mostly rules out going to local meetings. I'm lucky if I get any lunch.'

216. A lone specialist may not feel very welcome:
'I feel uncomfortable going to (internal) meetings where it may be the first time that many of the consultants have met you.'

217. Some meetings have ceased to be relevant:
An oncologist no longer attends general medical grand rounds:
'I used to, but I gave up a few years ago because I found it wasn't helpful.'

218. Library facilities may be limited and inter-library loan costs are high and may not be funded by the trust. This is particularly a problem for those working in the community trust.

219. Only one team member may be allowed to attend a course because of lack of funds for CME in the community trust. This is perceived to be unhelpful for practical skill development or shared learning and team working.

220. While on study leave the work does not go away:
   'The downside of attending meetings is that work is piling up so there is a price to be paid — you've got to work a little bit harder for a while to catch up, so I don't let myself in for that pain unless I think it's really worth going.'

221. Funds may not be available or the cost may not be justifiable:
   'Last year they froze the budget.'
   'Some of these things can be frightfully expensive and that can be quite a deterrent.'
   Some of those interviewed looked for sponsorship to attend national or international courses or meetings.

222. Relevance may be difficult to assess prior to the course.

223. Obligation may outweigh expected benefit, for example, the consultant physician who attends a regional research meeting related to his/her special interest:
   'I went to show support for the meetings but felt it was a waste of time — the research was poor quality.'

224. An appropriate course may not exist in which case a consultant may arrange to visit a known expert in the field, or design a course that fulfils a need. College accreditation for such courses has proved difficult.

225. Some of these barriers may be overcome, depending on the importance attached to the activity, the nature of the barrier, the ingenuity of the doctors and dentists and the support they are given by others. For example, some rely on a range of non-trust funding sources, either partially or exclusively. This is particularly so in academic/research contexts.

226. Some constraints seem to present insurmountable barriers unless substantial changes can be made to workloads and work schedules, the division of labour and the ways in which organisations and professional communities value their medical and dental staff. For example, as other community trust professionals (apart from psychiatrists) find themselves caring for people with mental health and behavioural difficulties, so their need for appropriate CME in these areas increases. Community clinicians' work schedules may mean that lunchtimes are taken up with travelling rather than attending meetings; the needs of staff grades may be poorly catered for by colleges; and staff grades can find themselves shunned by consultants at meetings.

227. Where a constellation of constraints affects an individual clinician, participation in some activities becomes impossible. The combination of distance, family commitments, a non-welcoming atmosphere and a high workload makes the uptake of elective CME unlikely.

Concepts of CME/CPD

228. Among the interviewees, the initials and the term CPD was recognised by only a few, e.g. psychiatrists because it is used by their college; or by those who have attended education courses; or by personnel officers. A number asked what it stood for. Only one, a medical staffing personnel officer, distinguished between CME and CPD in terms broadly similar to those in the 1994 SCOPME working paper.[11] One consultant seemed to think of the terms almost in reverse, CME being broadly concerned with all aspects of medical education, while CPD related to the professional/technical aspects of a specialty. Most do not routinely use a distinction between CME and CPD in their thinking in this area.

229. The concept of, and commitment to, continuing education was endorsed strongly by participants in this study. Some see continuing education as a professional obligation, some see it as a prerequisite without which it would be impossible to do the job, and some view it as an endemic feature of their professional lives, something that happens in the course of doing the job. No one argued that continuing education is, in principle, unnecessary.

230. CME has become strongly associated with clinical specialties and the colleges' credits system — traditional CME. Collecting 'CMEs' is now part of the language. CME is also closely associated with particular forms of formal activity, such as courses, conferences and meetings, to a lesser extent with audit and hardly at all with informal activities such as case conferences, discussion with colleagues and direct patient care. CME seems to be thought of as a formal or semi-formal activity, which provides knowledge in *'digestible form'* and *'take-home messages'* or the acquisition of specific skills. The range of activities from which doctors and dentists acknowledge they learn is much wider, but does not seem to be included in the category *'education'*. The latter seems to have more to do with that which is delivered by a formal education system.

231. For some there is a strong contrast between CME and education/professionalism:
   'Professional people are continually being educated.'
   'I think CME has lost its way. CME and audit are managerial ideas. It's all tied up with the difference between humanity and technology, education and training, control and liberty.'

232. Some make a distinction between CME and continuing medical education, the former referring to the system and the latter to a more authentic, educational process:
   'You know that if you sign a CME form at a meeting it just gets thrown away. As long as you personally are doing enough continuing medical education then it's meaningless, it's just added bureaucracy to your day — filling in the little booklet.'

Keeping up to date

233. Keeping up to date is a core concept in CME. Doctors and dentists in this study understand the concept in different ways.

234. For some, being up to date is primarily about maintaining professional pride and position among colleagues:
   'You want people to come to you as a useful opinion. You don't want to be thought of as a member of the B team. If people are honest, that's the prime motivator.'

Reference
11. SCOPME. *Continuing professional development for doctors and dentists.* London, SCOPME. 1994.

235. Such professional pride could be maintained by keeping abreast of developments; not being left behind:
'Cannot allow yourself to slip too far behind modern developments and medical changes.'

236. But keeping up to date is also an aspect of professionalism:
'Part of your profession is keeping up to date.'

237. And part of one's obligation to patients:
'Don't want to be left behind for professional pride and satisfaction and also because there is the duty to my patients to be aware of changing ideas and philosophies.'

238. And a legal obligation:
'Then there's the legal obligation — to avoid getting sued because you're not up to date.'

239. And includes safe practice:
'Demonstrating that we are within the norms of the profession.'

240. A central part of keeping up to date is keeping abreast of change and development:
'It's making sure you keep abreast of developments, new breakthroughs, re-evaluations of old treatments and the discarding of things which are well and truly passé.'

241. Being able to use what is new in clinical practice:
'In my field of vascular radiology there has been a lot of changes..... The forum by which they become accepted clinical practice does seem to be people reporting their experiences and talking about new developments and the problems they have had.'

242. Assessing when the evidence is sufficiently strong to implement change:
'There is often a lag of some time before you read about favourable trials and the consensus becomes favourable and you actually know how to implement the results. The early trial results can be the freak results of enthusiasts — there is the problem of knowing when you should start doing something.'

243. Reassuring yourself that you have not been left behind:
'I go along to some things where I learn relatively little but what I do learn is that I am not out of touch because it's not until you get a state-of-the-art summary that you realise — well, that's OK, what I thought was state-of-the-art is still very much state-of-the-art. Nothing has happened that I didn't know about which has left me behind. A large part of it is a checking procedure that you haven't missed out on anything significant.'

244. Maintaining a sufficiently broad knowledge base:
'Making sure you are aware of the most recent research.'
'Have to keep up to date, not only for general medicine but have to keep up to date with developments in the medical field — transplantation and immunosuppression and with antibiotics in terms of diagnosis.'

245. Methods for keeping up to date include regular reading, teaching, grand rounds, practising medicine, and attending meetings and conferences.
'Have to teach membership candidates so I cannot afford not to be reasonably au fait with the subject and there is nothing like having to teach a subject to make sure you actually know it.'

'By practising medicine — being it, doing it, you learn as you go along.'

'One of the important groups of people in this who educate me is the juniors because the juniors are rotating between the various consultants. They're the ones who carry the pollen from one flower to another.'

'The grand round is quite a useful exercise and it does give an opportunity to keep up to date on a broad front.'

'I attend advanced courses every three years in reconstruction or cranio-facial surgery. This is an essential part of keeping up to date with where this field is at.'

246. For some, keeping up to date involves maintaining a position at the leading edge of research:

'I look for people at the leading edge of research — quality speakers, an update rather than a more general talk.'

247. Others stress the importance of the leading edge of clinical practice:

'It's about best practice for your patients and making sure you are up to date with that best practice. It's not research related.'

248. For others, keeping up to date is much more about a 'general standard' maintained through reviews and symposia, rather than contact with first presentation papers in clinical science:

'There's a difference between keeping up to the general standard of what people are doing which is the reviews and symposia and forefront clinical sciences — first presentation papers. To be brutal, you would say that the cherry stuff was the only one that was essential and gives you points and be prepared to fund it as clinical director and give people time off. It would be possible to fulfil all your points and not actually update yourself.'

The CME system

249. There was rather less agreement about the extent to which the present college-run system was the best way to implement continuing education in practice. In formulating their views, interviewees distinguished between the system as a whole and a number of its components: the points and credits system; the record of activities — log book/diary; the categories of activity; activities included or excluded from the category system; the contribution of the system to ensuring doctors and dentists are up to date; and the relationship between their own activities and the category system.

250. The CME system is seen as both a measure of providing continuing education and generating income for the colleges and other education and commercial interests:

'Can be a bit of a gravy train.'

'We look at it as continuing education but the college looks at it as continuing education and the stability of the college. They go to these business people and say —make us some money.'

251. Interviewees describe the purpose of the system in terms of keeping doctors and dentists up to date — particularly the laggards — as a means of accountability to the public, a response to possible government imposition and a way of ensuring trusts give study leave:

'Nobody gives a toss what we like. It was self-imposed rather than being imposed because otherwise I think it would have been imposed by government.'

'CME is important but how do you ensure that everyone is doing it? For the average doctor you can safely assume that he or she will want to, but what do you do for the laggards? How do you enforce it? And, I suppose, this is one way of going about it.'
'What you are trying to introduce is a system that will just protect people — theoretically because they have the points.'
'CME is to overcome some difficulties with trusts who were refusing to release people for study leave.'

252. The system is seen positively by some:
'Works if one is focused and debriefs oneself after.'
'Good thing — it encourages getting away.'
'I see CME as an important aspect of clinical work. It ensures that people do undertake some form of educational activity to keep them up to date.'
'I think CME is pretty good but the question still arises, how do you pick out the outsiders?'
'It maybe brings on board those who haven't bothered and makes them more involved than they have been in the past.'

253. But more negatively by others:
'College system is a joke.'
'Does it make patients any better going on CME? I don't know'.
'This is a professional career. Part of your career is keeping up to date. CME doesn't need to be formalised. It runs very well with people going to professional meetings related to their special interest, and we all keep up to date by going to numerous professional meetings.'
'CME, as set up by the Royal College of Physicians, measures process not outcomes and tends to create its own demands which may not be at all effective.'
'One concern I would have about CME is the part-timers. At the moment there is no pro-rata reduction. If you're part-time you've got to do the same CME requirements as a full timer.'

The categories of CME activity

254. A number of those interviewed considered the categories of activity included in the log books/diaries to be a valuable guide to the distribution and balance of activity doctors and dentists should try to achieve. But, for some, such a balance is considered inappropriate because their activity grossly exceeded that prescribed in the college system and reflected a pattern which, although highly skewed in comparison with the distribution recommended by the college, nevertheless represented their needs and the availability of appropriate activity. For example, a super-specialist's activity may be dominated by international meetings and membership of a national audit project; the activity of a lone specialist in a DGH, e.g. a dentist, may be skewed towards national and regional groups and conferences with an almost total absence of internal meetings.

255. Many commented on the limitations of the categories to encompass all the activities from which doctors and dentists learn, including patient care, informal discussion with colleagues, reading and preparation for teaching, particularly as some of these were claimed to be much more helpful than attending meetings and conferences. For some, the categories over-emphasised academic pursuits, e.g. lecturing and examining:
'I think the Royal Colleges have got it badly wrong in that it includes lecturing and examining as allowable activities. CME seems to be run largely by academics and people in power and it suits them to have what they do included in CME.'

The points system

256. Many interviewees acknowledged that they did not regularly complete their activity log books/diaries and that they found doing so irritating and irksome. Nevertheless, some do keep their log books/diaries up to date.

257. All those who commented on the points system said they would pursue CME activities in its absence.

258. Some consider having to record their activity as rather demeaning, professionally unnecessary, irksome and *'a farce'*:

   'Am I supposed to walk round with a diary and get people to tick it off and should I, as a consultant, have to get some secretary to say I was there?'

   Others consider such policing is a good and necessary thing, provided the scheme is simple to complete and straightforward to administer:

   'I think being policed through the college points system is a good thing but I recognise that it may not change those who don't do CME. It has got to be a simple scheme and a points scheme in a book is as good as anything and the college is just getting its act together on admin. So it's best to keep it simple.'

259. Many of those who argued that the points system had some merit felt this was particularly so for those who might otherwise not take part in CME activity, but they had not themselves changed their pattern of activity since the scheme had started. Two considered they had seen a change in the pattern of CME activities in their directorates since the scheme was implemented, although this was not monitored by the majority of clinical directors.

260. Some interviewees use the points system as a guide to the balance of activity they should achieve. In some instances this was felt to provide a positive incentive to include more external meetings and courses. Others felt obliged to gather an appropriate distribution of points even where they felt they were gaining little from many of the meetings they attended. One considered national and international meetings *'a waste of public money'* in terms of learning gain.

261. Many commented on the anomalies of the points system, for example:

262. **Inter-college inconsistencies**
   'The royal college of surgeons counts reading but other colleges, e.g. pathologists, physicians, and anaesthetists, do not.'

263. **Potential for abuse of the system**
   'I know a lot of people, particularly if it's a meeting in London, they'll come to some of the lectures and then nip off and do a bit of shopping and then they'll come back and collect their certificates and home they'll go.'

267. **Attendance does not ensure learning:**
   'The bottom line is that you can take a horse to water but unless you are motivated to learn, to keep yourself up to date, learn new techniques, no amount of enforcement will work.'

265. **College conflicts of interest:**
   'The colleges are awarding themselves high allowances for their own courses and not granting such generous CME allowances to other bodies — it's a carrot to attract people to attend their courses.'

266. Broadly, rather fewer positive comments than negative ones were made on the colleges' role in the scheme.

267. Many of those interviewed formulated the CME dilemma in terms of how to police professionals:

    'CME is important but how do you ensure that everyone is doing it? How do you monitor the few who don't and are bad doctors, other than by their mistakes?'

    'How to enforce it? You want an open, non-fearful, non-punishing type of system. This is hard when you have people who know they can ignore the system and get away with it. But mostly they have their own internal carrots which is what you would expect with a system that produces autonomous individuals who can do it for themselves.'

    'It should be self-regulatory, but how do you regulate self?'

268. Some made suggestions for improvements:
    - Recognition of one's private study and reading;
    - Sub-specialties need to be recognised by the colleges;
        'CME process should be built into working time, not free time. There is a need for some slack in the system so that we can continue to educate ourselves';
    - Incorporate the internet-based material into CME;
    - Develop independent needs assessment;
    - Recognise as study leave visits to watch an expert using a particular technique;
    - More management and education courses;
    - Trusts should develop schemes for performance assessment;
    - 'If it was mandatory it might encourage those who don't go to many meetings';
    - Develop more local, regional meetings outside London;
    - Portfolios, as used by the nurses and general medical practitioners;
    - Reaccreditation:
        'I'm not very keen on the idea of having an exam every 10 years but I've talked to people who say, "How do I know the doctor I'm seeing is competent?" That's a good and valid question. Accreditation is the only way, but I don't know what happens if people fail the exam.'
    - Re-certification every 10 years:
        'I suspect re-certification is coming but I hope it won't happen in my lifetime.'
    - Strategy for CME:
        'It is the duty of the trust to ensure that consultants working in their organisation do continue their medical education.'

Organisational response to CME/CPD
Funding
269. Funding for CME varies between the three trusts involved. Most doctors and dentists in the DGH considered funding for CME to be generous, although they were unaware of the precise figure available. A sum of £50,000 per year is set aside centrally, i.e. approximately £625 per head per annum. The budget is not devolved to directorates and is not allocated on an equal shares basis, although costs incurred by individuals are monitored.

270. In the teaching hospital it was acknowledged that funding was less generous. A figure of £300 per head per annum was mentioned. The budget is devolved to directorates, included, unspecified, in another budget heading and not separately identified, as yet. Thus spending on CME reduced funds available to directorates for other things, as one

clinical director complained. Nevertheless, doctors in the teaching hospital had not been refused study leave on economic grounds, but they recognised the need to fund international meetings from other sources. These other sources seemed readily available and included special trustees, drug and equipment manufacturers, income generation, research and travel funds and personal monies.

271. Funding in the community trust is more problematic. Having recently merged two trusts and incorporated a mental health service from an acute trust, the community trust has yet to agree an overall funding strategy for CME. A figure of £25–50 per head per annum was mentioned as the sum available prior to the establishment of the single trust. While consultants seem able to access drug company funds to supplement what is available from the trust, staff grade doctors are more likely to have to identify very low or zero cost courses.

Organisational support and influence

272. Trust officers acknowledge that CME is an important matter about which the trusts should both take a view and have a strategy. But, for the most part, beyond such arrangements as postgraduate centres with their traditional role in CME, there is little evidence of a strong organisational role in CME. Nevertheless, there are elements of a developing organisational perspective, for example:
   - Reviews of CME being carried out by an associate director of medical education with each clinical directorate, to ascertain what activity is being undertaken and how it relates to directorate developments;
   - Developing links with nurse education and development;
   - Bringing together for educational purposes interests which may have been separated by the directorate structure, e.g. cardiology and acute medicine;
   - Recognition of the needs of new consultants, particularly preparation for their management and teaching roles;
   - Recognition of the isolating and compartmentalising effects of increasing specialisation;
   - Recognition of the need to revitalise audit.

273. Plans to provide regional college outposts in the teaching hospital will also have a local impact, as will moves for specialties with national and international reputations to become national CME providers.

274. The integration of CME with organisational policies and strategies is substantially missing in the three trusts involved. In some instances a clear separation is seen between the two — 'CME is not a trust or clinical directorate matter, it is a matter for the college and the individual clinician.' Other interviewees recognised the limitations of such separation, but also pointed out that the mechanisms to bring about change were currently absent, e.g. peer review, mentoring, appraisal, job plans, integration of audit with management.

275. In practice, CME is driven by individual clinicians and their commitment, interest and enthusiasm, within a provider led system. The result of this is that the trusts have no mechanisms for recognising educational needs, and individuals have no trust related routes through which they can channel needs they identify, apart from scanning what providers have to offer. For example, when a directorate structure is modified in ways that require specialists also to take intermittent generalist roles they may have abandoned some years ago, the trust has not recognised the need to provide generalist updating, not could the specialists involved find appropriate external generalist courses

and activities. Recent consultant appointees who find they have been poorly prepared for the scope and diversity of the roles they have to adopt also find that these educational needs are not recognised by the trust nor readily met from easily accessible CME courses on offer through familiar channels.

276.   While the community trust has an ambitious change and organisational development agenda, and is devising a trust-wide education and training strategy, developments to date have been focused on the establishment of agreed consultation and negotiating machinery. Nevertheless, the clinical director in mental health is reviewing job plans with consultants with a view to identifying training and development needs on a more structured basis.

277.   While the teaching hospital has easy access to a postgraduate and academic library and the DGH has a postgraduate centre with a library, the community trust does not have a clinical tutor, nor a postgraduate centre with a library, but does have access to these facilities in the local DGH. Nevertheless, plans are being made to provide library facilities in the community trust, but working across 500 square miles makes access problematic for many peripatetic staff.

Discussion

CME/CPD as we found it

278. On the evidence of the interview material, CME is being pursued by all the clinicians involved, for a wide range of reasons and purposes. While many exceeded — some by a very considerable margin — the levels of activity suggested by their royal colleges, a small number were finding it difficult to achieve the suggested levels in some categories. In a few instances, patterns of activity have broadened since the colleges' points systems started, but for most clinicians, what they do has not been substantially influenced by the system.

279. The term CPD is recognised by only a few doctors and dentists in this study, but the concept is acknowledged more widely. There are clinicians pursuing activities beyond those defined by specialty-specific interests, such as management and education. There are others who recognise their need for such additional expertise and there are those who espouse a more holistic concept of 'education' and 'profession' around which they have built their approach to medical practice in its widest sense.

280. CME is described by clinicians in management positions as, in theory:
    - A matter between individuals and the colleges;
    - A joint responsibility between the trusts and the colleges; or
    - A joint responsibility between individuals and the trust.

281. In practice, descriptions of CME reveal that CME is influenced by, and influences, relationships between individuals and a range of significant others, including colleges, trusts, directorates, departments, colleagues, patients and families.

282. The CME relationship between individual clinicians and colleges is perceived in a number of ways:
    - Ignored by some;
    - 'Them and us,' the CME system imposed by them and set up as a form of surveillance;
    - An irritation, but broadly complied with;
    - A good thing for persuading others to pursue CME but not necessary for me;
    - A way of making money for the colleges;
    - A necessary first step to ensuring clinicians keep up to date, on which further arrangements might be built;
    - A framework which helps individuals structure CME activity.

283. The CME relationship between clinicians and the trusts is largely characterised by the provision of variable levels of funding, from none to what is regarded as generous. Debates are beginning to surface about the balance of financial responsibility between individuals and the trust. While a culture of taking study leave is well established in the teaching hospital and the DGH, such a culture is considered to be absent by some clinicians in the community trust.

284. Trust managers recognise that clinical governance is likely to have implications for CME, but this aspect of the relationship has yet to be given considered attention.

285. In none of the trusts is CME/CPD managed by the trust through such mechanisms as business planning, quality, risk or human resource management.

286. The CME relationship between individuals and their directorates varies. While clinical directors see it as part of their responsibility to provide the right conditions for clinicians to meet their CME needs, this does not amount to a directorate CME policy and strategy. In the teaching hospital, budgets are devolved to directorates but are not earmarked. Spending on CME therefore reduces spending on other things.

287. CME has an impact on colleagues, through the benefits of dissemination of lessons learned and experience gained, although this is rarely done systematically. But colleagues may also have to provide cover for individuals on study leave.

288. Patients experience the benefits of improved practice as a result of CME although the evidence for this is not strong.[12] Patients also experience delays and cancellations when procedures are postponed and clinics cancelled when doctors and dentists take study leave.

Benign community neglect

289. The milieu in which CME/CPD takes place can be characterised as one of benign community neglect,[8] which provides space for practice communities to develop patterns of activity best suited to their growth and development. For individual members, learning is an inevitable consequence of participation in these activities. Through such participation, individuals are able to define and pursue a self-directed and individually tailored curriculum and become increasingly full participants in the community, i.e. increasingly competent and expert members of the specialty.

290. As the interview material and the model indicates, such benign community neglect affords participants access to a range of sites where medicine in its varied forms and versions is practised. Different versions of medicine are practised at the bedside, in the clinic, laboratory, seminar rooms and conference hall, but all are aspects of medical work. At these sites, practice communities display, rehearse, revisit, exchange, debate, challenge and, in short, make and remake, produce and reproduce medical knowledge in all its practical, theoretical, social, political and ethical forms. Through CME clinicians participate in these practice communities and thereby maintain and develop identities of increasing mastery, i.e. they learn.

291. The interview material and the model show some of the ways in which clinicians secure access to a range of practice communities through a mixture of choice, obligation, preference and interest and how learning occurs through engagement in activities at a range of sites of professional community activity.

292. The patterns of activity described by doctors and dentists in this study suggest that characterisations of CME as ad hoc and dominated by fact gathering in lecture format[13] fail to take account of the breadth of formal, informal, internal and external activities in which clinicians participate and through which they learn.

293. But the model is an ideal process and community neglect is not always benign. As the interview material shows, the process of participation in practice communities can be disrupted in many ways, some more severe than others. Such disruption can take a number of forms.

References

8. Lave J, Wenger E. *Situated learning: legitimate peripheral participation*. Cambridge, Cambridge University Press. 1991.

12. Davis D, Thomson M, Haynes R. Evidence for the effectiveness of CME. A review of 50 randomised controlled trials. *Journal of the American Medical Association* 1992; 268: 1111–1117.

13. Brigley S, Young Y, Littlejohns P, McEwen J. Continuing education for professionals: a reflective model. *Postgraduate Medical Journal* 1997; 73, 23–26.

Disrupting participation in practice communities
Ignoring salient features of participants' identities

294. Particular features may become salient as a result of organisational change, e.g. reconfiguring clinical directorates or by individuals changing relative positions in specialities, trusts and families. Isolation, defined in various ways, can engender a number of needs that may not be recognised and which organisational arrangements, or their absence, may frustrate.

295. In this study doctors and dentists alluded to isolation resulting from:
   - Geographical distance;
   - Heavy workloads;
   - Responsibility — the buck stops here;
   - Competition with colleagues for resources;
   - Sub and super-specialism;
   - Lack of the feeling of belonging;
   - Being out of mainstream career development pathways.

   Such isolation restricts opportunities for participation.

Imposing systems and purposes extrinsic to the core values and principles of the practice community, i.e. patient care

296. In the face of such an apparently unstructured arrangement as benign community neglect, it is tempting to impose structure and organisation, often for reasons of public accountability. The risk is that such systems divert energy and attention from the core values and purposes of the practice community and that the systems' objectives becomes goals in themselves. The CME points and credits system is one such. Collecting points distributed across a range of activities have nothing intrinsically to do with patient care. While the espoused purpose of the system may well be to improve patient care through CME, its immediate and practical goal is the accumulation of points, and that is how it is perceived by many clinicians. In response to the system some clinicians do things which, for them, are 'a waste of public money,' e.g. attend conferences from which they feel they learn nothing. Others skew their activity to bring it into line with the points system, but out of line with the ways in which they best learn.

297. Such a system is perceived by many to be other-directed and other-regulated rather than fostering self-direction and self-regulation. A number of clinicians justified the system on the grounds that it was put in place to persuade 'the laggards' to keep up to date, but, it is argued,[14] their needs require separate arrangements.

Lack of resources to enable increasingly full participation

298. Time is the main resource that career grade doctors and dentists need in order to participate in an appropriate range of practice community sites and activities. As many of the clinicians in this study emphasised, time is a precious resource in short supply. While many rely heavily on reading as a major means of keeping up to date, the irony is that finding or making time for reading is particularly difficult and is often snatched from other social, personal or family activities.

299. Time given for study leave is not equitably distributed across the career grades. While consultants may have a minimum of 10 days per year, some staff grade clinicians have only five. But during staff shortages, e.g. unfilled posts, consultants can find picking up the additional workload eats into study leave allocations. Study leave is not necessarily protected time.

Reference
14. Asbjörn Holm H. Quality issues in continuing medical education. *British Medical Journal* 1998; 316, 7131, 621–624.

300. While time may be made available, it is not always useable because of the way work schedules are organised. This is a particular issue for some community trust staff grade clinicians who have to use meeting time to travel between clinics and home visits.

301. More broadly, time required to travel depends on the location of meetings. For those in provincial locations, regional venues waste less travelling time than extra-regional or London meetings.

302. As with postgraduate education, time for continuing education and professional development is not always seen as an investment by trust managers, but rather as either an 'entitlement', which has to be accommodated, or an encroachment on service demands.

303. Funding is a further necessary resource to enable participation. Budgets available for CME are not always clearly identified and known to the clinicians who draw on them. In the absence of such clarity, rumour and guesswork abound, with very different accounts being given of the ready availability of funding by different people in the same trust. Experiences of seeking funding also vary. In the DGH no one considered funding to be problematic, except for staff grade doctors, for whom the position had recently improved. On the other hand, in the community trust, views and experiences varied considerably, from *'We didn't do any external CME last year because the budget was frozen',* through *'We are often expected to fund half ourselves',* to *'I usually manage to get what I want for courses'.*

304. Access to different funding sources varies. The teaching hospital seems to have a wider range of sources on which clinicians can draw.

305. The availability of, and access to, library and information resources vary depending on where you work. The most comprehensive facilities are available to doctors and dentists in teaching hospitals, through the adjoining medical school. But lack of funding for journals in the library and no access to the Cochrane Data Base were mentioned as limitations. Clinicians in the community trust who work at some distance from a DGH may have no easy access to a library. They may make use of other facilities intermittently at the teaching hospital or in London, but have to pay personally for inter-library loans.

306. In general, the allocation of resources to facilitate access to practice communities and their activities seems to reflect an educational version of the 'inverse care law' — those who need most get least or those have most are given more. There seems to be an implicit assumption, built into the way resources are allocated, that those who do less glamourous, more routine, less ground-breaking work have less need of continuing education and professional development.

Denying access to provider decision making

307. Many doctors and dentists in this enquiry acknowledged being often *'disappointed'* by courses and conferences they attend. Their hopes and expectations were not realised. While many providers now routinely request feedback ('happy sheets') after meetings, only a few seem to follow up comments in order to find out precisely why delegates were not satisfied. Some do design their courses around gaps in knowledge identified from self-text MCQs completed by clinicians. A number of clinicians commented on the variable quality of what is on offer and an apparent absence of effective quality control involving them.

Impact on specific groups

308. DGH dentists are few in number and might be thought to be particularly vulnerable to non-benign community neglect. Yet despite the fact that there is little of relevance to them going on in their hospitals, they have links with local regional and national networks of colleagues in which they can participate. But distance, and the absence of daily informal contact, does make it difficult to maintain the momentum in activities such as audit.

309. Community dentists share the general absence of a continuing education culture and lack of resources for CME with other colleagues in the community trust. But as the client groups seen by community dentists change, so do their CME needs. Community dentists are now seeing fewer children and more elderly people and people with special needs. As a result, a process of sub-specialisation is emerging, but CME providers have not yet responded to this need.

310. Staff grade doctors in the DGH vary in their perceptions of CME and the opportunities open to them. Those who have recently taken up staff grade appointments and are working towards or have just passed college examinations, are largely satisfied with CME arrangements and are involved with some internal and external CME activities, but not at the level of consultants. Nevertheless, there are examples of more experienced staff grade doctors who work in isolation from consultants, feel marginalised in the trust, blocked in their careers and neglected by the colleges.

311. In the community trust, staff grade doctors, particularly women with young children, find it difficult to 'get their CMEs'. They, too, feel marginalised, that their particular needs are not recognised and that consultants shun them at meetings.

312. Particular concern was expressed about the appropriate involvement of part-time clinicians in CME.

Conclusions

313. Enhancing participation in practice communities can best be achieved by working to reduce and eliminate the causes of disruption to participation. More proactively, enhancement can be developed through the relentless and single-minded pursuit of the communities' core values uncontaminated or distracted by other goals and objectives, in ways which ensure that the core values are realised in practice.

314. This study has found that most doctors and dentists involved have developed, or are in the process of developing, *'a habit'* of continuing education tailored to their needs, involving engagement with a range of sites of practice community activity. Much of this activity is central to continuing education and professional development, although 'invisible' to the CME system.

315. Taken as a whole, against the background of all that medical and dental work entails, the clinicians' patterns of participation in CME/CPD have a scope, coherence and structure which, while not amounting to rational planning, is far from ad-hoc. Trusts and royal colleges facilitate, but sometimes disrupt, such engagement and participation. All those involved should be given credit where credit is due.

Appendix A: Methodology

316. The purpose of this study was to understand the ways in which career grade doctors and dentists in three NHS trusts choose, carry out and evaluate CME/CPD activities. In-depth interviews were conducted with 64 doctors and dentists and one personnel officer from a teaching hospital, a district general hospital and a combined community and mental health trust. Dentists from a small department in another DGH were also included. Individuals were interviewed in their clinical and managerial roles.

317. The study was qualitative and used in-depth interviews and critical incident technique (an interview technique that asks participants to describe events which have gone well and events that have gone not so well). Single interviews of 30–45 minutes per participant were requested. 'In-depth' would therefore be constrained by what might be expected of participants in this time. The view of the following groups were sought in the numbers indicated:

Teaching hospital consultant doctors	28
District general hospital consultant doctors	17
District general hospital consultant dentists	5
District general hospital staff grade doctors and dentists	5
Community trust consultant doctors and dentists	8
Community trust staff grade doctors and dentists	1
Personnel	2
TOTAL	**66**

Specialties included:

Medicine	12
Pathology	7
Anaesthetics	6
Surgery	6
Head and Neck	5
Imaging	3
A&E	3
Paediatrics	7
Psychiatry	4
Cardiology	2
Oncology	1
Orthopaedics	1
Liver Services	1
Dentists	6
TOTAL	**64**

318. The total includes 16 clinical directors, one director of medical education, one clinical tutor and three medical directors and one personnel officer.

319. A number of loosely structured interview schedules were prepared for different groups of participants; doctors and dentists, clinical directors and clinical tutors and directors of personnel. These schedules were devised to include the broad themes and objectives of the enquiry.

320. Requests for participation were sent to a teaching hospital, a district general hospital, a community and mental health trust and a district general hospital with a dental department.

321. A sample of potential participants was drawn up to broadly represent the numbers of doctors and dentists in each directorate. All dentists and staff grade doctors and dentists were included.

322. Of these interviews, 63 were face-to-face and 63 were audio-recorded.
All audio-recorded interviews were substantially transcribed, i.e. between four and six A4 pages per interview of largely verbatim material.

Methods of analysis

323. A form of content analysis has been used to identify themes, sub-themes, issues and concerns addressed in the interviews. Each member of the enquiry team worked on the material from the interviews he/she carried out, but a number of transcripts were examined by all three interviewers as a check on consistency.

324. Material in relation to individual interviews was collated, e.g. activity, reasons for participation, perceptions of effectiveness, and notions of CME and CPD.

325. Relationships and interactions between themes were examined, e.g. how specific activities were selected and their effectiveness assessed.

326. The material was examined to identify potential findings, e.g. individual activity profiles and their relationship to the doctor's or dentist's position in the specialty and/or to working patterns and interactions in the department.